CrossFit is anabolic and kinetic and can be enjoyed by anyone.

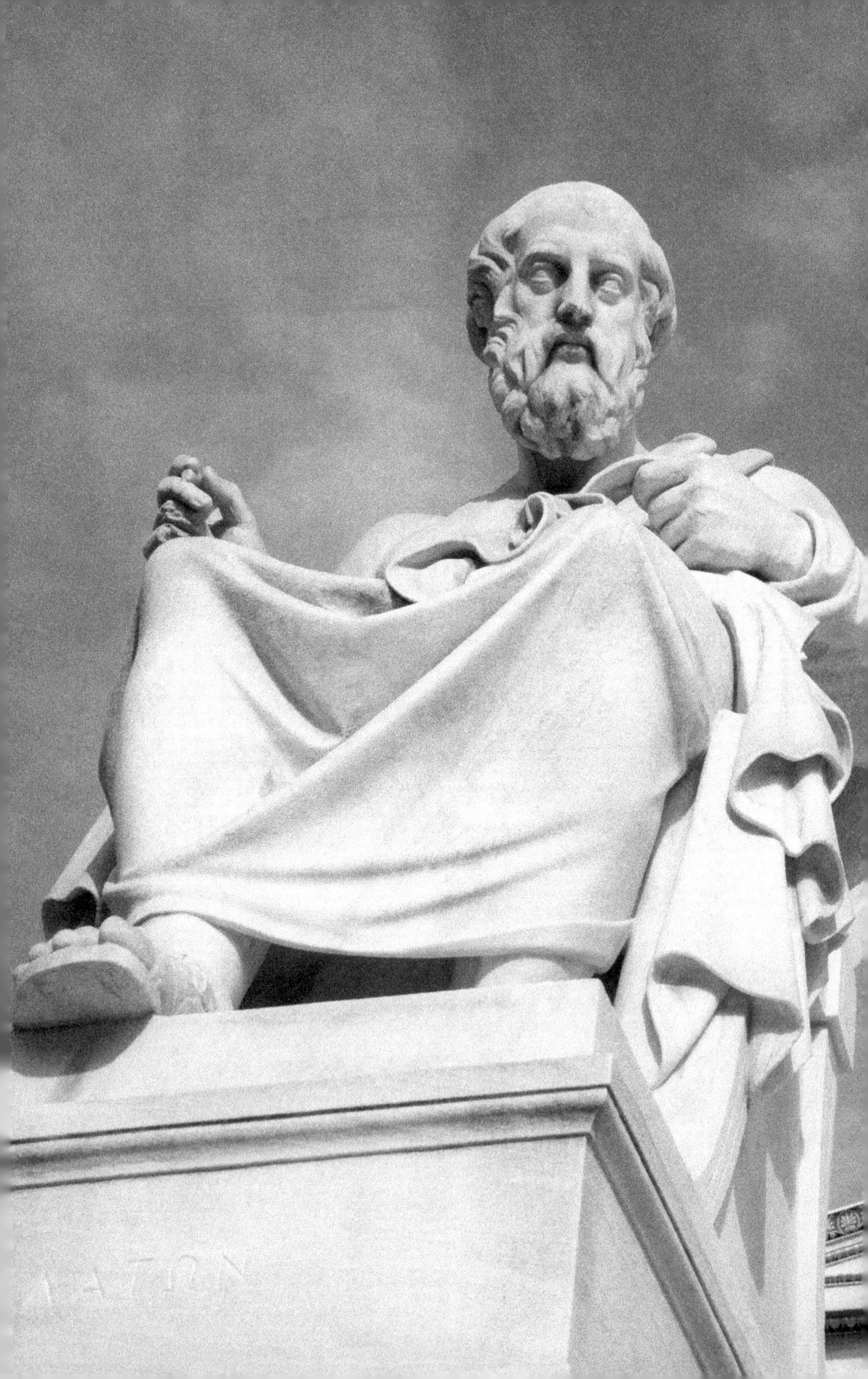

"Overpower. Overtake. Overcome."
—Serena Williams

"When a resolute person steps up to the great bully, the world, and takes him boldly by the beard, he is often surprised to find it comes off in his hand, and that it was only tied on to scare away the timid adventurers."
—Ralph Waldo Emerson

"You gain strength, courage, and confidence by every experience in which you really stop to look fear in the face. You must do the thing which you think you cannot do."
—Eleanor Roosevelt

"Courage, sacrifice, determination, commitment, toughness, heart, talent, guts. That's what little girls are made of. The heck with sugar and spice."
—Bethany Hamilton

"When I think of fear before starting something, I write down my thots. When it's all over and I've succeeded or failed, I think about the initial fear for a moment, laugh about it, then forget about it and burn the note."
—Anonymous

"We can easily forgive a child who is afraid of the dark. The real tragedy of life is when people are afraid of the light."
—Plato

"Never be afraid to try something new. Remember, amateurs built the ark, professionals built the *Titanic*."
—Unknown

"Everything you want is on the other side of fear."
—Jack Canfield

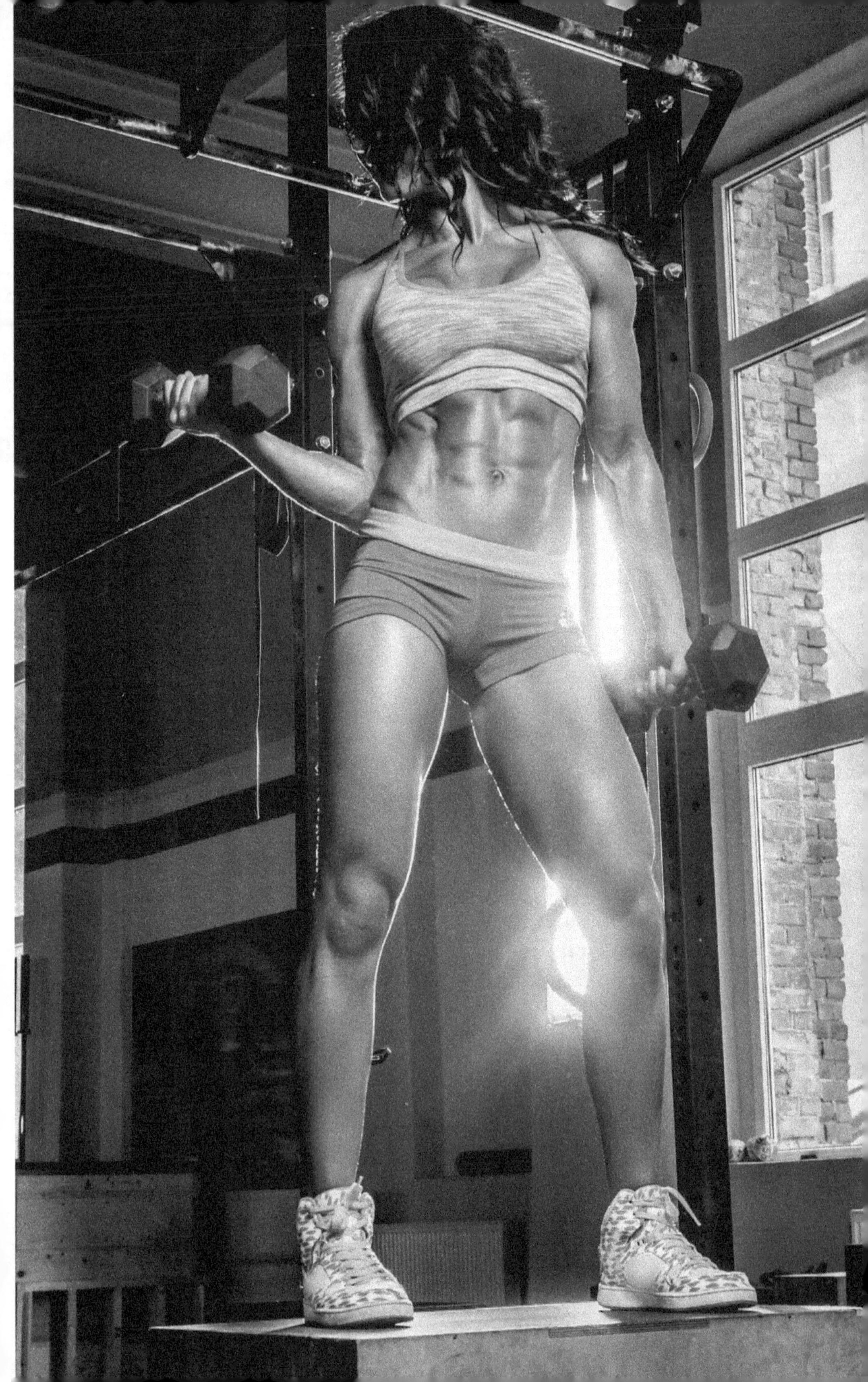

61 IS THE NEW 41

CROSSFIT YOURSELF TO HEALTH & WELL-BEING

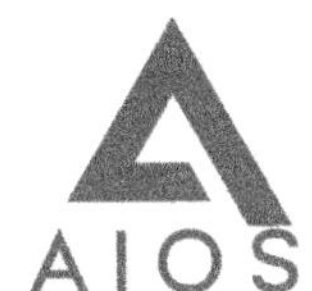

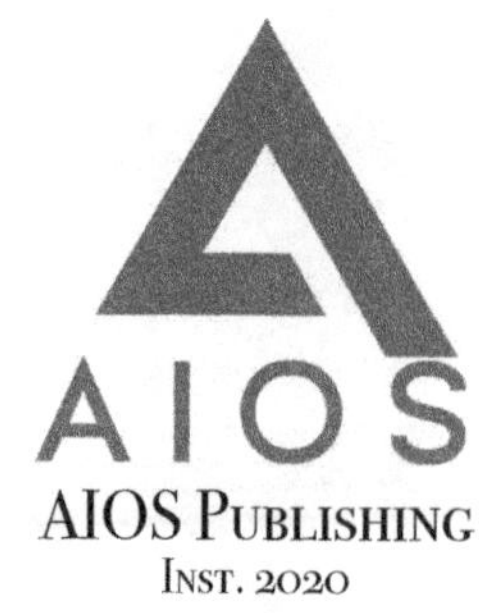

AIOS Publishing
Inst. 2020

Published in America by AIOS
AIOS and its colophon are trademarks of AIOS

Library of Congress Control Number: 2021936308

Print ISBN: 978-1736272671

DISCLAIMER / SUBMISSION

This book and its eBook version are works of nonfiction. The information offered within these pages is for educational and entertainment purposes only.

We assume no legal liability whatsoever for its content, usage or implementation.

The contents in this book are not intended for use as medical diagnoses, prevention, and/or treatment of any health issues.

If you follow the directions in this story, you'll pro'ly have fun, feel fantastic, and wanna do it again tomorrow. And then share it with others. Yes, it's addictive.

AIOS-P20210701
First release: The First of July 2021

for Coach Patrick Higgins
Mentor, Coach, SoulCare Guiding Light, Friend

for John
Brother, Friend, Forever Partner in Crime and Mischief

and for You, fellow CrossFitter!
Friend, Colleague, CrossFit Professor of Exercise

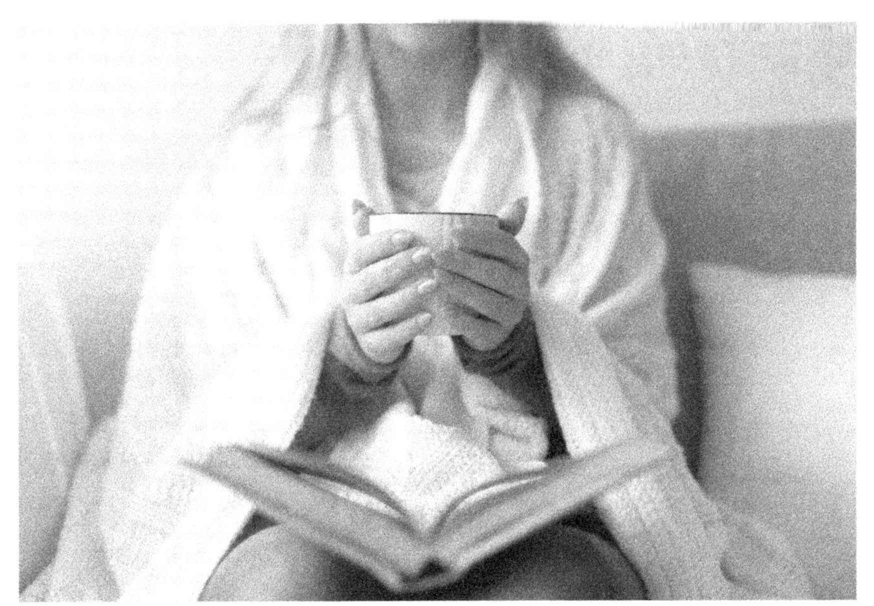

Table of Contents

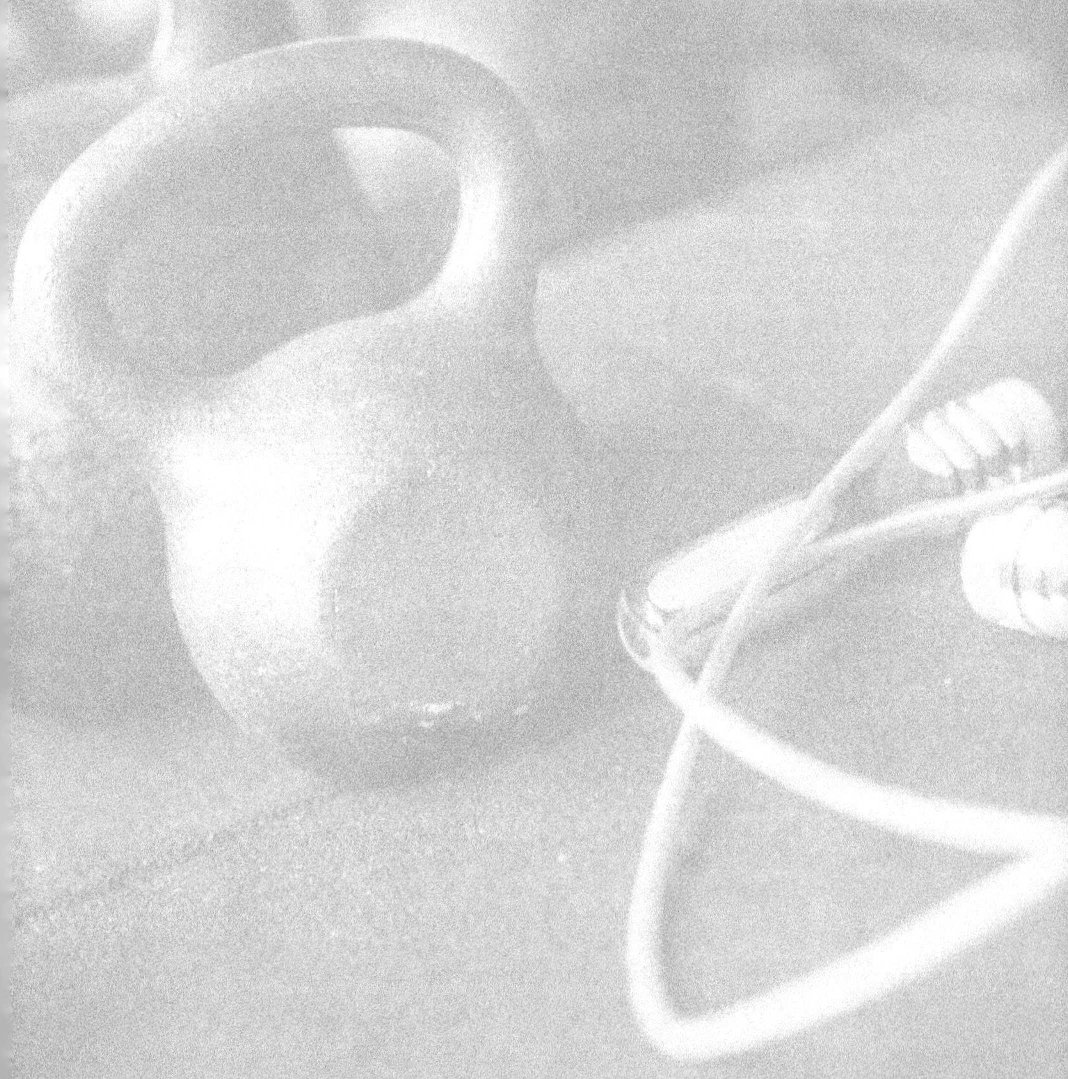

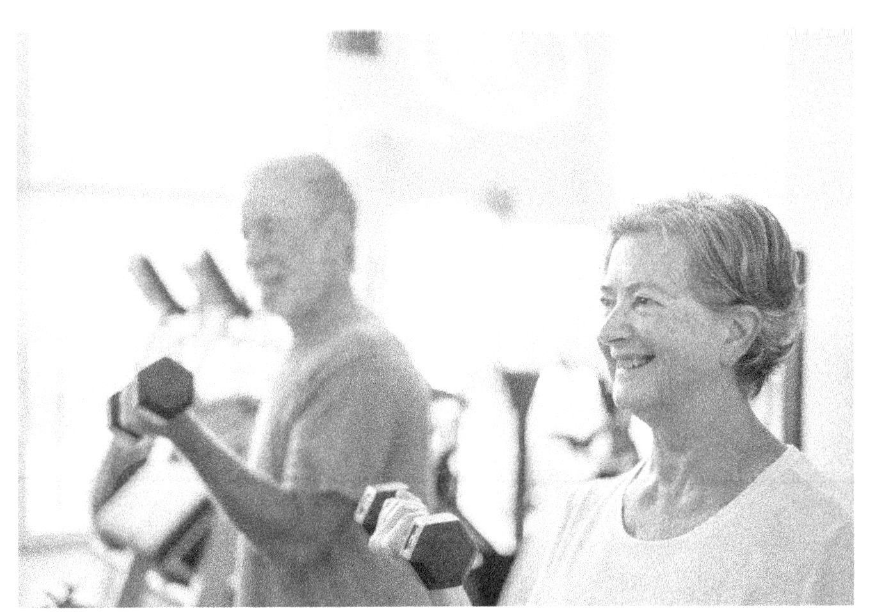

0 Hello, CrossFit!

"There is no try, only do."
—Yoda

Yoda is sitting on my shoulder right now, trying to find a comfy position. He twists and jerks my head thissaway and thatta way so it doesn't interfere with his hyperbolic gestures, rustles his nearly thousand-year-old hand-woven smock, adjusts his light sabre so if it goes off it won't lop off my ear. Or cabeza.

The Jedi Master smacks me on the back of my head, says, "Take dictation, you will. Talk, you will not. Only listen and absorb. Much wisdoms of The Force follow, they will."

While Master Yoda prepares me to receive his bold wisdoms so I can transcode them into proper English for you, I am thinking: *How do you introduce a book that's more than its title suggests?*

Kinda like $e = mc^2$: an infinitesmally small amount of matter, when broken apart, yields a massive amount of energy, much more than was promised.

This isn't some self-help book about CrossFit. Yoda don't do self-help books. Yoda tells stories of adventure and action, sprinkled with the uncommon wisdoms of Jedi and The Force.

Yes, *wisdoms*. It's a Yoda thing.

$150 A Month!? Are You Kiddin' Me!?

61 Is The New 41 is a kinetic story of a journey to becoming a better you by using CrossFit as your new *exercise* routine. I pray this story inspires you to make a huge change in your life and crossfit yourself to health and well-being.

By the way, you don't have to be 61 years old to enjoy this book. It's really for anyone interested in starting their exercise routine and getting healthy for life.

As I explain in Chapter 1, crossfit is now a verb. Relax, it was Yoda's idea, same as it was with his term "potato-couching." But that's a story for Chapter 4.

Yoda tells us to put away childish things and begin at the beginning: as I explain later in this chapter, there's a huge difference between exercising for fun and fitness, and training for various levels of competition. This story reveals how to understand that difference and embrace *exercising*.

Besides, most people do not want to train at an elite level. They simply wish to get fit by exercising, using CrossFit as the medium. And they don't want to spend an arm and a leg doing it.

I want you to know this up front: CrossFit costs an average of $150/month for unlimited workouts and full access to a CrossFit box (gym). Add more if you do private exercise or training sessions.

For some, this is excessive, especially since non-CrossFit franchise gyms across the US are charging only $9.99/month for full-access memberships. Hey, but they ain't CrossFit.

Please do not be discouraged by price before you engage this story. I also suffered sticker shock when I stepped into my first CrossFit box. They wrote down the price on a piece of paper and slid it across the table. After chatting up the lead instructor and his partner, I found a workable solution (read: I got me a darn good discount).

My favorite coach said it was also the best and most important investment I would ever make in life. Putting it that way made me see it in a different light, and I then placed very high value in this new investment in my life, my future.

A Story Conjured Out Of Necessity

The original concept for this story was simple: do an article for Austin Heaton for his cool website, HeatonMinded.com. Austin even suggested my sending the article to CrossFit CEO Eric Roza.

Respectfully, the article grew wings of its own and morphed into a 220-page storybook of inspiration. Thankfully, Austin understood and encouraged me to continue on this new path.

In this story, I discuss what you can expect from CrossFit, how it affects your body, and many of the untold hidden benefits from doing it consistently. A lot of those gems come directly from people who have taken a leap of faith and dived into CrossFit. Their stories are moving and inspirational and are the soul of this book.

In Chapter 4, I also share my own 27-step program for starting CrossFit, which is sort of a long-form Betty Crocker recipe for lifelong success. Honestly, I pro'ly could've just used Chapter 4 as a one-chapter book on how to start CrossFit.

Yeah, but it wouldn't have been as fun and adventurous without the other chapters of anabolic spice and kinetic energy.

My aim in sharing this story with you is to show you that CrossFit is not the scary training program you've probably heard about. It is not all about training like an Olympic athlete 24/7 for years, only to burn out at age 30.

My coach related an anecdote: "I talk to these people all the time and they tell me how they see the elite CrossFit athletes on tv, all bulked up. And they say they don't wanna look like that or have to train five hours a day like them.

"I tell them, 'You watch NFL football on tv, right? And you love tossing around the football with your son, right? Are you saying you won't do it anymore just because you think you'll turn into a massive NFLer?' At that point, a lightbulb goes off in their mind and they see they point: you can also just exercise in CrossFit and not become a muscle-bound athlete."

Although CrossFit, Inc. does not currently promote this, you can *exercise* instead of train, and scale down your routines to get as much out of each workout as you want and your body needs.

My dream: CrossFit will become a worldclass *exercise* program and a primary key to greatly improving your health and well-being. If ever there were a fountain of youth, CrossFit is it. Just look at Yoda: he's been doing it since . . . over 800 years ago.

On The Verge Of Total Collapse

Are you currently a little tired, with achy and slack muscles and joints? Do you have difficulty bending over to touch your toes or pick up your grandchild? Are you slow to wake up in the morning, even though your delicious breakfast awaits you in the kitchen? Are you lacking in motivation, in general? Feeling lethargic?

Do you wish for something better?

I was there a year ago so I know how you feel. If you will please trust me here, I will guide you from feeling like crap every day to a whole new sensation of well-being. For the moment, I need a few small things from you: your precious time, willingness to listen, and eagerness to make some important changes in your life.

Like I said, I was there and it was sheer misery every day: going to bed at all hours of the night and day, sleeping poorly and waking up every hour in a sweat or dry as a bone, having terrible nightmares that delivered the same message to me, drinking a six pack of beer upon waking up, stepping out on the patio for a Marlboro Blue Menthol, looking down at my fat belly and shaking my head in disgust, walkin' in pain to the next room, eating three McDonald's double quarter-pounders with cheese (hold the pickles) or a cold pizza, chasing breakfast with two Dr Peppers, plopping down in front of the big-screen tv and bingeing on Netflix, Amazon Prime and every movie and tv show I'd bought on Apple TV.

My biomarkers screamed at me each time I had them measured: high triglycerides, high blood pressure, low testosterone, low thyroid, low B12 and D3, high cholesterol, and just about every bad "high" and "low" you can think of.

My primary-care physician kept telling me: "You have to stop eating so much at once, you have to stop consuming refined sugars, you have to stop eating processed carbs, you have to stop drinking alcohol, you have to stop [FILL IN THE BLANK].

With him, it was about "stop this, stop that." And he meant well and his message was clear.

My subconscious took a different approach: it told me to start something positive. Start getting up early and walking. Start eating some fruit or oatmeal for breakfast, start drinking a lot of water during the day, start going to bed early. Start . . . something *positive*!

Very soon, all the "starts" began telling the "stops" to piss off and head on down the road. Sometimes, it's all in how you see and value something. *Starting* something was much more positive for me than *stopping* something else.

Like many of my peers, I was only 60 years old, in worse shape than my 87-year-old father, but not quite as bad as mom. She passed away at age 57, her ashes scattered over a special place.

I was on the verge of total collapse and was stuck in an insular world I created for myself, perhaps a coccoon to secure me while I decided my next move. My recurring dream was being a pile of ashes just before a hurricane came a-huntin'.

What a wonderful life I'd had up to that point and the bitter irony was that I'd spent much of it assisting and helping others . . . but not myself. And since I'd isolated myself and kept my issues to myself, no one knew how I was feeling.

Kinda like how I treated cars in my youth: ran them ragged without ever changing the oil. I burned up and melted many an engine and was now repeating this bad habit in a gruesome way with my own health.

Shedding An Old Skin

Here's the beauty of the whole process: your new reality emerges from the seemingly impossible dream, thus leaving in its wake the old plan that drove you to ruin. There's much to be said for shedding an old skin and starting afresh.

A mystery of life: sometimes one's own story, as it is being conceived and written, becomes the single path that leads you to health and well-being.

The key is to allow your *subconscious* to guide you, be your mentor along the way, because your conscious self (the bus driver, I call it) cannot be trusted at the moment. It is the entity that drove you over the cliff, even though warning signs were posted all along the way.

Who in their right mind would trust a driver like that? Many people, evidently. I discuss your subconscious in great detail in Chapter 13, and how to use it as your mentor in starting and maintaining your CrossFit routines and also in your daily life outside of exercise.

What follows is a strong, positive story that, with the assistance of my subconscious, wrote itself as I slowly clawed and climbed out of the grave I'd dug for beautiful me.

Maybe yours is a similar story, filled with the highs of marriage and children and the lows of bad health and death.

Regardless, we share the same goal: improve our health and well-being. With that said, I carry on eagerly and bravely.

Changes You Can Expect From CrossFit

Today, every BabyBoomer is over the age of 55 and fast approaching 61. More than ever, that silver tsunami of 75 million souls needs to listen up:

I'm sure you'd love to learn about how CrossFit can transform you into a new you. In addition to discussing the state of the art of well-known neurotransmitters involved in producing positive feelings, I will share with you the obvious changes in how you will ***feel*** once you begin your CrossFit journey and exercise consistently.

CrossFit incorporates many different exercises and routines, all done at different intensity, speed, duration and number of repetitions. The human body responds differently when you move slowly for a certain period of time. It responds in other ways when you jog, run, or sprint for short and long distances.

It reacts in different ways when you pick up weights and hold them in certain positions for a certain period of time, or push and pull them for a number of repetitions.

Mostly when you exercise hard over an hour, say, your body reacts by ensuring you have enough energy and chemical resources to maintain that slow but sustained level of working out. It also rewards you with that euphoric high, encouraging you to continue your great work.

At the end, you will feel a definite change in how you feel. It will be a tingly feeling, one of euphoria that last hours after you stop exercising. You will soon crave this upbeat feeling, thus pushing you into your next workout.

Seemingly, this perpetual energy violates the First and Second Laws of Thermodynamics, and that's okay because it works within you and makes a better you. Please be a renegade and violate those silly "laws" en route to feeling great.

If you move at a faster pace for that hour, your body reacts by adding new and different chemicals and it calls up different chemical pathways and cascades. All of these complex reactions ensure that your physiology will keep up with your movements during that hour and ensure you are well rewarded.

It also will further build your strength and stamina, and improve your endurance. Your mental health also will improve: cognition increases, allowing you to process information and to think better and faster and more efficiently. Your ability to control your emotions, self-regulation, improves, too.

In Chapter 4, I discuss in detail something you're gonna need to try: "metabolic biohacking." And Chapter 12 has some cool facts and thoughts on your gut microbiome and how exercise improves its functions. In fact, every subsequent chapter has new information that will stimulate and inspire.

Please be patient and keep reading. . . .

Your Body Has A Factory Of Cool Pharmaceuticals

The feeling of euphoria and a special "high" is due to a combination of special neurotransmitters in your brain, working in concert with chemicals outside the central nervous system.

Those of you who have a disdain for marijuana and its various cannabinoids may be surprised, if not disappointed, to learn that your brain has endocannabinoids (ECs) and specific receptors for them. Their effects on your brain are very similar to those produced when you smoke pot, although the concentration of ECs is much less.

We may not have the hundreds of different ECs contained in a typical marijuana plant (leaf, stem, root, and the various products produced external to the plant), but we definitely possess enough to evoke the various "highs" and euphoric sensations we feel during and after a moderate and intensive workout.

Runner's high is due primarily to our ECs, dopamine, endorphins and oxytocin (and stuff we haven't discovered yet). Dopamine is also known as the "reward molecule," because its pathways are involved in producing reward-driven behavior and seeking pleasure. Endorphins, a portmanteau of "endo + morphine" act mainly as painkillers.

Ever heard of the hormone oxytocin? It's also produced in the brain and released by the pituitary gland. When you show feelings and actions of love and lovemaking, it enters the bloodstream and soon enhances your orgasm, and produces other sensations and feelings.

Studies years ago linked it to bonding between a mother and her newborn, but recent work shows that it encourages bonding in men and women without babies. The molecule is involved with touch, tactile sensitivity, sex and lovemaking, and bonding among group or tribe members.

The EC/dopamine/endorphin/oxytocin euphoria and sense of bonding and closeness you experience will be greater the more you exert yourself during workouts, especially when you do interval bursts of activity. You rarely, if at all, experience euphoria and that high when working out slowly and for short periods of time.

Your own body will let you know when you've hit upon the right zone of exercise, and will reward you. A paradox: holding poses in yoga for long periods also can evoke that euphoric high we see in moderate or intensive CrossFit work. Perhaps it's not a paradox at all, just another side of your body's internal reward and pleasure system.

We don't really know enough about all the body movements and activities that produce this euphoric high. For now, we simply know that they work to make us feel like a million bucks when we exercise.

The body knows that you are exercising it and wanting to build it into a better you, so it gives you little treats to encourage you to continue this exercise. Your body has a mind of its own, and it wants to be fed, as well.

It loves the sensations of climbing, jumping, bending, twisting, running, pulling, pushing, gripping, grabbing, etc. It loves even more the sensations that accompany those exercises.

Essentially, when you exercise, you are pleasing both you and your body at the same time. It also loves those periodic bursts of activity that appear to be just as important as the regular exercises.

By working out using the myriad exercises in CrossFit, you are creating and building and shaping new neurochemical and biochemical cycles and cascades. Many of those contribute to that euphoric high.

Others simply build a better, stronger, faster you who is more flexible and has better endurance. Of course, there're many other benefits we've yet to discover.

This is why so many people, who have yet to discover the benefits of exercise, turn to drugs like heroin and cocaine for this same high. Unfortunately, their artificial highs are often too much for the body, and they crash and burn.

You don't have to resort to an artificial high. I suggest you continue reading this story about CrossFit and discover your own path to evoking that natural euphoric buzz. It's something you can feel every day of your life, and do it in moderation so you don't get burned out.

Beyond the buzz, you will experience a new level of fitness, a new you, and a new way of life and living.

The Absolute, 100% Proven Benefits Of Aerobic Exercise, Punctuated With Intensive Anaerobic Bursts

My personal journey has included every type of exercise out there, and I've done many of them in combat situations. I love running long distances for many hours at a time. I love hiking up mountains at night. I love swimming in the ocean (long as the sharks keep their distance from me!). I love great sex. I love all forms of movement, some extreme.

The best form of exercise that mimics that total movement I love so much is CrossFit. Period. No other gym routine does that.

Yes, and it makes sex much better. What's better than sex?

To me, it's that euphoric high you get from doing intensive

exercises, both aerobic and anaerobic. And it's the great feeling I get when seeing the positive results of my blood chemistry, and the definite changes I witness in how I look. I discuss these in detail in Chapter 4.

As if those reasons weren't enough, please consider this short list of "hell-yeahs!"

Exercise . . .

1. Gives you energy and increases your resistance to fatigue, meaning that although your body is working harder when you exercise, over time, you feel less tired than you did before you started working out.
2. Makes your muscles stronger, improving your ability to do many different active tasks, and increasing your independence, as you are less likely to need help with physical tasks.
3. Makes you more flexible, increasing the variety of physical activities you can do, whether they are directly related to exercise.
4. Improves your endurance, meaning you can continue to be physically active for longer periods of time than you can when you don't exercise, without straining yourself or feeling uncomfortable.
5. Makes your body more efficient at physical tasks, meaning you can do them with less effort, and feel less tired afterward, than if you don't exercise regularly.
6. Reduces your risk of injuries: lower-back problems, flexibility issues, muscle pulls and strains, tendon/ligament strains and tears.
7. Helps you to manage your weight and will assist in losing weight if you are overweight.
8. Decreases your risk of cardiovascular disease.
9. Reduces your risk of type 2 (adult-onset) diabetes mellitus.
10. Significantly lowers symptoms of depression and will help manage those symptoms for those who have it.

11. Decreases the effects of aging through improved functioning during regular tasks of everyday life.
12. Assists people overcome other addictions.
13. Helps you to get a good night's sleep and assists in assuaging sleep disorders.

Now that you know the end result of your journey, all you need to do is start at the beginning, fill in all the blanks, have fun and . . . ***exercise!***

Start *Now* To Overcome These Common Health Issues

As we pass mile-marker 60, a lot of funky things happen to our body, and sometimes we don't even notice them. Mine sorta crept up on me, as you read earlier, and when I did notice them, it made me mad!

I was mad at myself for getting into this mess and not doing something positive about it. I was beyond rock bottom. In fact, I crashed right through it and discovered a whole new kinda hell that had no defining features, not even proper nomenclature to describe and define it so I could make sense of it.

All I knew was that I had become a piece of crap of absolutely no use to anyone.

After my 60th birthday, I noticed my skin first: it was kinda dry with tiny wrinkles. I'd never had bad skin. Ever. My genes were top notch, but not even they could fight against my neglecting my body all those years. It's as if I went to bed looking as I had at 36, then woke up as a 60-year-old turd.

There was also an invisible enemy I had yet to discover and deal with: trillions of microbes inside my GI tract, in direct communication with my brain and all other parts of my body. It was my body's ultimate demon, something science had yet to recognize, define, study and deal with.

Most people who are not athletic or active during their life don't have good bones, muscles and joints. Mine were in excellent health despite my general state of disrepair.

For others, though, the bones and muscles, ligaments and tendons get loose and lose strength and resiliency. Tendons, when suddenly pulled into action, rub over nerves and pinch them into a lightning-hot pain that stays for weeks. Muscles pull and tear easily, and are very slow to heal.

Depending on your level of activity and general health, your metabolism slows about 5% each year after age 30. That means you must eat less, especially at one sitting, and be more active. For those who are largely sedentary, this means that you gain more fat and lose muscle mass. Though not well known or understood, your gut microbes are very likely the cause of some, if not all of, these issues.

The GI tract is less active, thus creating more blockages in your intestines. The transit time for food to pass increases, thus leaving toxic foodstuff inside your intestines much longer than normal. It's worse if you don't drink much water, and especially bad if you drink alcohol and smoke cigarettes.

We also tend not to eat enough fiber, which causes more constipation and the slow sloughing off of our protective mucus lining in the colon. This in turn leads to leaky gut, allowing microbes to enter the bloodstream and cause all manner of health issues.

The heart still pumps away even at age 100, but if you don't take care of yourself, it will fail. Heart disease is on the rise in the US, mostly due to a poor diet and alcohol/drug abuse. Now, too, we know its health is influenced by your gut microbes.

As we age, though, the arteries and veins, arterioles and venules, and capillaries all begin to lose their physical and chemical integrity. Also, their tensile strength decreases and our pipes and tubes harden, primarily because of calcification.

When you exercise, you are gently mechanically stretching and contorting your arteries and veins, arterioles and venules, and your capillaries. The idea is to keep them nice and stretchy so they convey blood, lymph, etc. much better and more efficiently.

Moving each day causes a mild stress on your cardiovascular pipes. Our body responds to these thousands of tiny stressors by ensuring our cardiovascular system's health is well maintained.

The connective tissue and its components that hold our pipes together and also gives them tensile strength is continually upgraded and replaced as needed.

Example: when you lift a barbell over your head, you are stretching hundreds of different cardiovascular pipes because the movement forces the arms and shoulders to pull and extend and elongate.

In turn, all the pipes within the muscles and other tissues elongate with the movements. You are effectively exercising and improving the health of your cardiovascular system and thus decreasing your risk of stroke and heart attack.

Bummer: your sex life can take a nose-dive if you aren't healthy. Diabetes causes erectile dysfunction in men. In women, multiple issues cause the vagina to become dry and unable to produce the mucus necessary for comfortable sex. Vasogestion is also a problem with women.

Your body's immune system, 70% of which is modulated by microbes in the gut, is most important in your 60s and beyond. Unfortunately, its response to harmful stimuli decreases and it does not protect you the same as it did in your youth, and your gut microbes have a big say in this decline.

If you aren't in good shape, your level of happiness and well-being will drop considerably, mostly because of the added stress. That stress weighs heavily on your mind, causing depression and anxiety, among other health issues.

Memory loss is a horrible condition, and it occurs more in those who aren't physically and mentally active. Even though your brain is capable of producing new neurons and other associated support cells, lack of exercise, age, and a sedentary life will inhibit growth. No one wants early onset dementia. The gut microbe-brain axis is compromised during lack of exercise. Microbes may be responsible for some, if not all, neurodegenerative diseases.

Good news: when you start your new CrossFit program, some or all of these issues will lessen considerably or disappear altogether. You will also increase your body awareness, self-respect, self-esteem and so much more.

My own grand life now is proof that this process works, even starting from a hundred feet below all the crap that served as the mile-thick foundation under rock bottom.

It feels like I wrote this story as a lifeline to pull myself from the abyss and to surface again, with a new life and a different purpose and direction.

Your good fortune: this story is also especially for you, a new source of inspiration and energy that will change your life for the better.

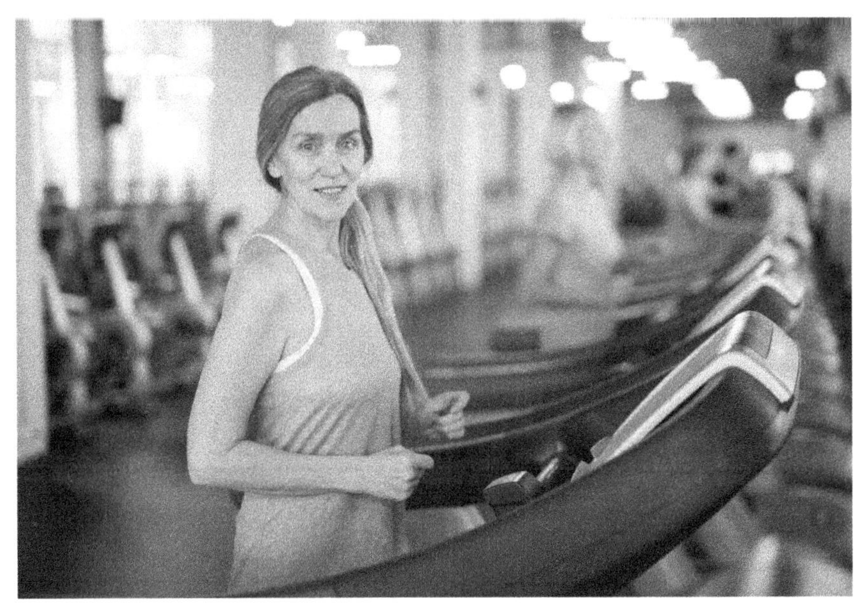

1 A Plucky Foundation

"If you have time to whine and complain, then you have time to find a solution."
—Chris Winter

First things first: for those of you wishing to transform yourself into a new and healthier you, I'd like to introduce you to ***CrossFit!*** Currently, CrossFit is branded as high-intensity interval training that includes many elements of Olympic weightlifting, powerlifting, gymnastics, calisthenics, yoga, running, and many other types of exercises, leading to a whole-body workout that builds muscles, increases endurance and produces a natural feeling of well-being , all of which create a healthy and happy new you.

The daily workouts are known by crossfitters as Workouts of the Day or WODs. WODs usually go an hour at a time, with yoga and stretching done in between workouts. You can scale and tailor your workout to suit your fitness goals.

Do not be scared off by all this new stuff! As I discuss soon, you don't have to become the elite CrossFit athlete you see on tv or in documentaries. I am suggesting a whole new line of CrossFit routines that center around *exercising*, and not training at a high level.

Please absorb the information and take a deep breath, perhaps many. CrossFit is all about skill, knowledge and efficiency, and being able to sustain those in a healthful way over a long period of time, not just a few years. You will, in time, learn all these new concepts and put them to good use so you can develop a good exercise routine that will take you well beyond middle age.

But you must go slowly at first, so please listen and learn. I promise this: you will discover immediate use for this new exercise program. It will surprise you how easy it is to start, once you've dismissed the myths about CrossFit, those silly things that frightened you and kept you away from this fascinating way of life.

CrossFit actions are very similar to those you perform in your daily life: bending over, squatting down to pick up something, reaching way above your head, pulling something across the floor, pushing a load over your head, picking up bags of soil or rocks, running down the street to catch your cat, and the like.

CrossFit sometimes has you do these exercises very quickly or very slowly, depending on the WOD. The speed, acceleration, duration and repetition all contribute to a great workout, and the desirable after-affects will last well into the next day. Your muscles, joints, tissues, cells and genetic machinery will adjust to the new routine, and begin to build and strengthen.

Doing these exercises several times a week will greatly increase your flexibility and range of motion, so you can perform your normal daily duties with ease. After six months of CrossFit, I went from being a slug to a sprite young man again. Well, sorta.

Little did I know at that time that I would greatly increase my flexibility and range of motion of all limbs and joints. I'm still not as flexible as a yoga guru, mind you, but I can do everything I need and want in life, and do it with the body and physiology of a much younger man.

Two 70 year olds at my box have gone from looking like broken-down jalopies to limber and flexible 40-somethings. You will, too!

Presently, CrossFit is undergoing an overhaul, with the hope of attracting people who are interested in high-level training. There aren't that many people who wish to train at an elite level, yet the CrossFit brass seem to think there are. I say they're just plain wrong.

They've not yet adopted my idea of attracting those who wish to *exercise*, not necessarily train. Let's hope this book encourages those at CrossFit Headquarters to consider my suggestion and revamp the overall program to include the rest of us.

The world of CrossFit is so much more than what I reveal here, but I couldn't possibly explain it in a book. I encourage you to read this story, absorb it, let it diffuse around your beautiful mind, and then begin your journey to health and well-being.

If a picture is worth a thousand words, then a visit to your new CrossFit box will be a *Magnum Opus*, made just for you.

Current Books On CrossFit Do Not Sell Well. Why?

Initially, I wanted to design and build a book that would introduce you to CrossFit and encourage you to try it out, see how it fits you and your current lifestyle. I wanted to write you a story about CrossFit, not simply throw dry facts and statistics at you.

My aim was not to create a self-help book, either. Nope, there're too many of those on the market and even though they may sell in the beginning, they're not much use in the end.

I've seen all the books on CrossFit there are. They don't work for me as a new crossfitter, but I love the stories they tell. They are more like biographies than CrossFit books.

Considering there are 15,000 CrossFit boxes around the world, plus millions of would-be crossfitters who wish to exercise and not train, statistically I would expect 100,000-500,000 people, minimum, to buy a good book on CrossFit.

Current books on CrossFit seem to appeal to die-hard fans who follow the sport religiously. The reviews of each of these books strongly suggest this.

It is safe to report to you that, based on the statistics, there are no good books on CrossFit that assist a beginner to successfully enter the world of CrossFit and to exercise or train.

My aim is to change that. And maybe this story is just that change.

Putting it simply, you can't effectively write an instructional book about CrossFit no matter how many step-by-step instructional pictures you use. There're many books out there that try to do just that, though. The statistics don't lie and they paint a somewhat bleak image of the state of the art in producing useful books about CrossFit. Makes me wonder why people continue to produce these books.

My prayer and wish are simple and humble: This is *not* a self-help book. It is a story that transcends any books on exercise, weightlifting, CrossFit, etc.

I pray this story will grow into a respected narrative on how to transform your beautiful life, using CrossFit *exercise* as both the medium and the message.

Many People Think They Need Self-Help Books

Self-help books are a big seller on Amazon. As of this writing, the #1 book in the Self-Help category is *You Are a Badass: How to Stop Doubting Your Greatness and Start Living an Awesome Life*. There are more than 25,000 reviews over the past eight years. Wao.

When you examine the negative reviews, you see the dark underbelly of the book, the true shortcomings that anger people and cause them to dismiss it outright. I won't elaborate further here.

Another popular book in that category is *Self-Love Workbook for Women: Release Self-Doubt, Build Self-Compassion, and Embrace Who You Are*. Last I checked, its sales rank on Amazon was 32, which means it sells about 18,000 copies a month. Many reviewers like the book and praise its content, so maybe it is right for them in some important way.

I read this book. Some parts I loved! It does read more like an "activity book," as one reviewer pointed out. The suggestions are sometimes too general to be of any real use to someone in the throes of depression or a break-up.

Me? I would seek the advice and counsel of a living, breathing Licensed Clinical Social Worker (LCSW), rather than a bestselling self-help book authored by an LCSW.

We all need human contact. Books and other study and learning materials have their place in our lives, yes, but there's no substitute for a live human who guides and mentors us. Same with CrossFit!

Generally, when people look for self-help books, they are very eager to learn about something important to them, something they feel they cannot learn on their own or from trusted family, friends or colleagues. A great example is the huge popularity of Don Miguel Ruiz's Toltec Wisdom Books.

His beautiful stories seek to explain how/why we begin as wise ones and somehow allow society to scam us that it knows better about us than we do. I read all his books and love them like oxygen. Those of us who read the Toltec Wisdom series are clearly looking for answers to the many questions we ask about our own existence and purpose.

Those beings who control us use powerful propaganda and slick manipulation to steer us away from our own wisdom. Those same powers tell us to follow and believe in them, not in our own thoughts, ideas, beliefs. Such is the power of so-called self-help books, pushing us to seek answers outside ourselves.

I have a simple message for you: You have inside you all the answers you need to enjoy a wonderful life. You may not know all the details about something, but you certainly have the framework to understand it.

Most of us are too insecure to strike out on our own and learn something from scratch. So we turn to the easiest thing available: a book. Or a YouTube video! Anticipation mounts as we research the book(s) we think we need and want. And when we find something that looks promising, we quickly buy it.

A friend who works at Amazon in Seattle told me most people don't spend much time researching. They look for the first few books on the subject on Amazon and click BUY NOW. That's impulsive. Perhaps even desperate.

It belies the fact that people are very eager for knowledge, and they wanna cure what ails them or learn something entirely new and fascinating. This reveals the wonderful side to us humans: we thirst for knowledge and self-improvement, and find ways to quench that thirst!

Unfortunately, 99.999% of self-help books that describe how to do things are discarded very soon after they're purchased, because they do not deliver on their promise and also because those books are not tailored to fit each person. You don't see book reviews written long after a self-help book is read. They're typically written when the reader has just received it and glanced through it. I'm generalizing but with accurate data.

Self-Help Books Fail For Many Reasons

The main one is that the reader cannot figure out how to use the information to their advantage and get something useful out of it. Almost all the self-help books I've read or glanced over come with lists.

Many people I've talked with hate lists. They don't write them let alone use them, so lists are useless to them. These people are report not being goal oriented. They live in the moment and see what life brings them.

Self-help books don't address these special issues like an LCSW, good therapist or counselor would.

All self-help books should come with a warning label, one that states that self-help books truly do require the in-person assistance of an expert, as I state above. Simply reading the material somehow does not translate well when looked at, stared at, read silently or aloud. It just doesn't work for most people.

Paradoxically, self-help books largely fail, but they do manage to sell millions of copies. Some are definitely bestsellers, but they are certainly not *bestreaders*, mostly for the reasons I outlined above.

If someone came out with different versions of a self-help book, one for each personality type out there, then it might work.

Good News: *61 Is The New 41* Is Not A Self-Help Book

It is a story about a journey to crossfitting yourself to health and well-being, with a few tried-and-true suggestions and hints, plus testimonials from crossfitters who've done the work you're about to start.

Just so you know: I've read dozens of books on exercise and CrossFit. None of them worked for me. It took my getting off my butt and visiting a CrossFit box to learn how to engage in this fascinating and important means of exercise. At that point, I wanted to write this story and share it with you, with the hope it will inspire you to do as I did: get off my duff and start a whole new life and lifestyle.

If I have just insulted or maligned self-help books, please accept my apology. I only meant to share with you the importance of doing things in person with a mentor, coach or instructor. Besides, you can always stop the action to ask them a question and get immediate feedback. Those self-help books don't receive questions, let alone provide answers.

See someone in person to get valuable lessons and feedback on your actions and movements.

And feedback about your attitude, in general.

You just can't get that from a book, no matter how well styled and presented. Or well intentioned.

CrossFit, In A Nutshell

Like I said, this book isn't just a book about CrossFit. It is a brief introduction on how to begin a new exercise regimen, using CrossFit as the medium.

61 IS THE NEW 41 isn't simply a catchy title, it's a way of life, a new philosophy, a different way of thinking about health and well-being. It could've been titled *41 IS THE NEW 21* and marketed to a younger crowd.

It is also a moving story about CrossFit and features the journeys of brave souls who shared with me their personal struggles, both physical and mental.

CrossFit is, delightfully, the stickum that binds us in a common passion and pursuit of a more healthful life and new lifestyle. Some may call it our reason for existence.

There's a cool French word for that, isn't there? *Raison d'être*, methinks. Yeah, that's it: CrossFit is your new raison d'etre. Now all you have to do is spring into action.

How This Story Begins

Essentially, this story is a revelation about how we humans often live an ordinary life, hit a brick wall at some time and reach a breaking point that welds our shoes to the floor, preventing us from escaping.

We are now stuck and can't get out, so we pause to consider where we landed and how badly messed-up we are, make a plan to get out of the world of crap we put ourselves in or were thrust into.

Success or victory comes when we steer that plan to a well-coordinated goal or a personal triumph over what we thought was an impossible obstacle.

Not sure how to structure it at first, I called on a few trusted friends. They unanimously suggested I lead off with how I came to discover CrossFit, what it's done for me, and how it has shaped my current life so I could write this book and inspire others. Mind you, I'm nothing special: average height and weight, decent looks, easy genuine smile, good athleticism and coordination, reasonably intelligent. So I figured if an average human like me can do CrossFit, surely other 61ers and younger people will, too.

> "There's a huge difference between training and *exercising*."

61 IS THE NEW 41 also features the personal journeys of CrossFit Games winners Dave Hippensteel and Armando Besne, both of whom are over 60 years old. And also the journeys of Rachel, Lynda and Bobby, who choose to *exercise* and not train like Dave and Armando.

All of their stories should motivate you to consider how CrossFit may benefit you after 60, even if CrossFit is the furthest thing from your mind.

Exercise Or Train? There's A Huge Difference!

Remember: you have a choice whether to *train* like Dave and Armando or simply *exercise* a few times a week for fun and fitness. Like average Rachel, Lynda and Bobby.

It is up to *you* whether you make CrossFit sport (exercise) or labor (training). Training is what athletes do every day to prepare for competition. It takes considerable time, effort, money, energy and a 100% commitment. That, my friend, is hard labor.

When I was in the military, I used to train relentlessly for combat missions. Grueling, backbreaking work every day for years. All that was hard-core training and execution, not simply exercising. Talk about a labor of love.

Exercising is a way of life, too, but it is a slower-paced activity, sustainable over many years. It's an entirely contrasting dedication with less burden on your mind and body.

You still get that wonderful feeling of well-being, but without the 24/7 dedication and devotion for high-level CrossFit training. It doesn't produce any gold medals but it does assist you in sustaining your workout routine over the long run.

To me, living a really healthful life is like earning a gold medal every day.

That elite level of training, i.e. chasing gold medals, takes a toll in the long run. You can't do it forever. However, you can exercise until you die.

Witness Exhibit A: Mat Fraser. He genuinely burned out at age 30, after taking the CrossFit title five times. The cost to him and his family and friends was enormous, though this was downplayed in the media. I pray he now will enjoy exercising each day for the rest of his beautiful life.

Me? I wake up every morning and do some kinda exercise. I couldn't *train* every day and feel well, much less pull myself outta bed. Other "slack-athletes" feel the same as I do. Note: the term is in no way derogatory, so don't go there. Thank you.

Now that I think on it, the term "slacklete" suits me just fine. Please consider this neologism my small contribution to describing those of us who *exercise*. Still, calling recently retired Mat Fraser a *slacklete* is a bit of a stretch, so let's not tell him.

I hope you'll appreciate why I decided to focus on exercising, not training. This is something you can get into at any age and do for the rest of your life. If you do it correctly, your injuries will be few. So far, I've only had a minor shoulder strain, and that's mainly from sleeping wrong some nights.

CrossFit helped me cure that issue by aligning my muscles, tendons, ligaments and shoulder joint, and forcing them all to work together correctly. It was my own "chiropractic adjustment."

I'm proud to say that several enthusiastic and energetic non-competitive CrossFit athletes contributed their uplifting anecdotes to this story.

While they are not at the level of elite CrossFit athletes, they demonstrate that anyone can begin a journey into the realm of CrossFit, and enjoy it to its fullest without burning out. It starts with a spark that, with time and patience and effort, becomes a raging fire.

My wish is that CrossFit, Inc. CEO Eric Roza will recognize the need to give newcomers and current crossfitters a choice to exercise like I've suggested above, or to train. His current marketing efforts definitely do not work in the long run.

Several CrossFit boxes I contacted ceased being official CrossFit gyms because there weren't enough "elite" athletes who wanted to train at a high level. Now these gyms simply have ordinary people who exercise by following "CrossFit routines" but not calling them CrossFit routines since they're no longer affiliated with CrossFit.

Mr. Roza may reach his goal of getting 100 million people to do CrossFit in 10 years if he changes CrossFit's self-image, public persona, and approach to working out, i.e. recognizing that you can either *exercise* or train.

At the moment, CrossFit Headquarters is looking at it the wrong way and will continue to scare away those who wish to exercise for good health and well-being.

Most people, though, likely will choose to use CrossFit as a way to *exercise*. Once they start gaining strength and endurance and that euphoric buzz each time they crossfit, along with noticeable improvements in their overall health, they will tell ten friends, and they in turn will tell ten friends.

It becomes a geometric progression, the multiplicity of which is ten. That's huge, especially when it spreads quickly by the best advertising and PR in the world: word of mouth.

A Story Not Just For 60-Somethings!

Once again I pray that I have sufficiently embraced the beautiful thoughts and feelings of those souls whose stories now fill these pages, plus have done equal justice to the quotes and helpful thots by seasoned professionals whose wise words added spice to this story.

After having experienced their moving stories, either through emails or phone calls, I admire and respect them greatly, and hope you will, too. They still serve as great inspiration and energy for me as I continue my journey in CrossFit.

Honestly, this story is not just for those of us who've reached that special milestone: 61 years old. Or, as many now choose to view it, 41 years *young*.

There's a big part of me that wanted to write this book for *anyone* who wants to start CrossFit, but when I thought it through, I felt I needed to focus on those who probably needed it the most: my beloved peers.

By the time you reach 70 and 80, you most certainly will *not* be sitting in a wheelchair in an assisted-living facility, playing bingo and Old Maid, waiting to die.

You will be active on your own, flying among all those kids half your age, and implementing all those lessons learned over the decades, and the new ones you learned doing CrossFit.

What's more, you'll be sharing your wisdom with previous generations, a great gift.

Oh! Let's not forget that euphoric high you will get each time you exercise with your fellow CrossFit athletes.

My secret goal in life and wish for all: Transform CrossFit into the world's safest, most efficacious formula for *exercise*, one that produces excellent health and well-being for all. This new standard sets the example for all others to follow, and encourages everyone to improve and expand on it and to start a CrossFit revolution.

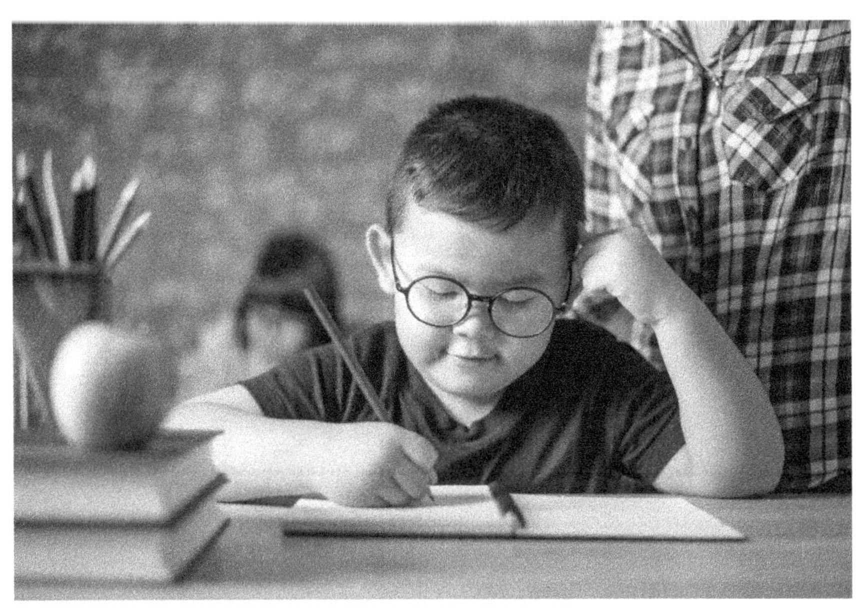

2

Humble Beginnings

"Move."
—Dr. Timothy Leary

This story, like all my literary and creative projects, has humble beginnings, although it flowed from crazy-big dreams and mighty wishes. After all, I live by the adage, "*Anything* is possible" and by my own rule: "Everything I do has a 100% chance of success."

As I mentioned before, it was originally designed as a series of interviews for an online article, featuring age 60+ CrossFit athletes, both seasoned veterans and starters like me. Then this covid thing happened and things began to evolve into something unexpected.

The last thing I wanted to do was produce a self-help book. As I said before, you can't write a self-help book about CrossFit.

My goal was to write a lovely *story* that would inspire people to pursue CrossFit as a new lifestyle choice, and to exercise their way to health and well-being.

A Special Birthday Surprise

I was still working on books, but everyone else was in panic mode, wondering if they'd have a job in a month. I felt bad for my friends and colleagues, so I kept quiet and pressed on with my own work.

No one was available to chat, let alone sit down and write their answers to my endless questions. Eventually, I got antsy and started calling people again, and managed to anger a few souls who were still out of work and in no mood to chat. Said a prayer for them and moved on. Again.

Soon, though, on my 61st birthday, on Thanksgiving 2020, people started calling and emailing me to discuss the project. In a very short time, it morphed into a journey that revealed hidden motives, desires, wishes and passions in the middle-aged athletes I had the honor of speaking and working with.

"Crossfit is now a *verb*. Use it wisely, spread it generously, add a few new definitions to it, if you will. In a few years, it may be as versatile, elegant and timeless as the term *f-ck*."

It was never meant to be a 400-page tome. I've read many of those by guys like Tim Ferriss, and I love them dearly, but I knew my audience of 60-year-old athletes wouldn't be sitting around reading such a book, regardless of how well it was presented.

As you'll soon see, these age 60+ kids don't do too much sitting. We boogie at many an opportunity, because we know age doesn't get any easier and time seems to zip by without our noticing.

A tiny revelation: in 2020, I read 405 books, all in the 300- and 400-page range. It was a self-dare, something I'll not do again, even at gunpoint, because the pages whipped by at a pace much too fast for me to enjoy well. I'm going back to my usual 300 or so books a year, a much more manageable pace for my schedule.

I'm pretty certain my friends—and I imagine you, too—do not spend that much time reading books, let alone 405 in a year. In this country, we are not taught or encouraged to read books.

Magazines and tv shows and movies of all stripe smack us in the face, scream for our attention, and keep it for decades.

This current book is for those consumed by mass media and entertainment, maybe a tiny story for those five or ten minutes on the potty each morning. Thank goodness it's also an ebook, so you can carry it with you wherever your iPhone or Android goes.

Please do not accidentally drop your phone in the toilet. Apple phones can withstand a good dunking down to 30 feet for a few minutes, so it's safe at the bottom of a toilet or pool. Dunno about Androids so good luck.

That's why I decided to binge-loop my boy Bruno Mars' *24K Magic* and *Perm* at 120 dB day in, day out and pen something short and powerful, a little book of inspiration I hoped would spark enough interest in you to find your nearest CrossFit box and give it a whirl.

If all you manage to do is read this baby, then I kindly ask that you absorb what you can and pass it on to a few 60-somethings in need of a physical and mental tune-up. And months of Bruno.

2020: My First Year In CrossFit

I did just that in June 2020, after a few months of Bootcamp at another local gym. It was a good warmup, Bootcamp, but not what I truly needed to get to where I wanted.

Besides, I knew from experience that you cannot simply do a few exercises for an hour then sit around for the rest of the day. I needed a shock to my system that would jumpstart each day and propel me into being at least moderately active all day. Bootcamp didn't cut it.

CrossFit grabbed me by the throat, squeezed really hard and hasn't let go since. Bootcamp just didn't provide all the necessary weight training I was looking for to make a better me.

All it took for me to engage and fully commit to getting healthy again was diabetic neuropathy in my feet from a sad case of diabetes I'd developed slowly over the years.

I was angry that my body was fighting me, and so I wanted to fight back and cure myself, if possible.

I'd been an athlete all my life and now was saddled with a box of broken bones, squishy out-of-shape muscles, and a seemingly incurable metabolic disease whose origin may have been in my own gut.

Through it all, though, I maintained a strong positive attitude and outlook on life. Attitude: how you see the world and react to what it throws at you are *everything*. Developing and maintaining a strong, positive attitude can turn you into a superwoman or superman. The choice is yours.

Me? I choose to see the world and everything in it in the most positive and constructive and optimistic ways possible. Even in the worst of times, trust me. I have always turned bad situations into a hilarious comedy sketch. That great attitude has saved my life a few times in combat situations.

Two years prior, I quit drinking alcohol and smoking cigarettes. Never much of a smoker, when I fell into disrepair I started "enjoying" that burn at the back of the throat from cigarettes and many a beer, sitting at tiki bars up and down isles in the Caribbean.

When I did US military and civilian special operations work, I never drank or smoked on missions. The job made certain demands and I complied.

After I left special operations, my smoking and drinking increased a lot, and it cost me $1,000 a month to maintain those two habits. Heck, I loved that "two-beer buzz" in the beginning. Thing is, I never stopped at two. I was, and still am, one who binges on just about everything. Things taste better when administered in large concentration all at once. It's that shock to the system that turned me on.

A nagging dissonant noise in my subconscious kept at me, begging me to make some lifestyle changes so I could live and play well into my 70s and maybe 80s. After years of neglect, I finally changed the way I looked at that two-beer buzz, discovered for the first time the underlying dissonance, and made those changes cold turkey.

I'm not sure how that abrupt change affected my gut microbiome, but it seems to have adjusted. Could be, too, that I created a whole new imbalance in my gut bacteria and other microbes. I don't know. It's still a work in progress.

And at the beginning of each month, I discovered I had an extra $1,000 dollars in my pocket. Woo-hoo!

Self-hypnosis worked well for me, thank goodness, and I still use it today, even for small things. It's all about how you view and value something.

My wish for you, dear reader, is that you become inspired to get off your hiney-bumper and crossfit yourself into excellent shape and a whole new life and lifestyle never before imagined, and see this mind-blowing way of life as your fountain of youth.

I cannot emphasize this enough: you do not have to train like an elite athlete to enjoy all the benefits of CrossFit. You can *exercise* your way to good health and well-being. The difference between the two also cannot be overstated.

CrossFit Is Now A Verb

Yes, my friend, "CrossFit" has been transformed into a verb: crossfit.

Use it wisely, spread it generously, add a few new definitions to it, if you will.

In a few years, it may be as versatile is the f-word, which has so many incantations I can't even recall them all.

Crossfit you, dude!

Oh, crossfit off, homeboy!

What the crossfit!? WTC?

Oops, not a verb but it sounds almost respectable.

Oh, baby, crossfit me! Crossfit me!

Admittedly, it may take some time for crossfit to morph into something as cool as the f-bomb. For now, let's enjoy it in its simplest form. Get to your nearest CrossFit box and crossfit yourself to great health and well-being.

My gentle advice to you: fasten your seat belt, hold on tight, and enjoy the short ride. Think of it as hopping on "Flight of Passage," the new Avatar ride at Walt Disney World, closing your eyes and just *feeling* the adventure.

cross·fit | 'krôs,fit |

verb

Engage in high-intensity fitness exercise that incorporates elements from many different sports, types and styles of exercises.

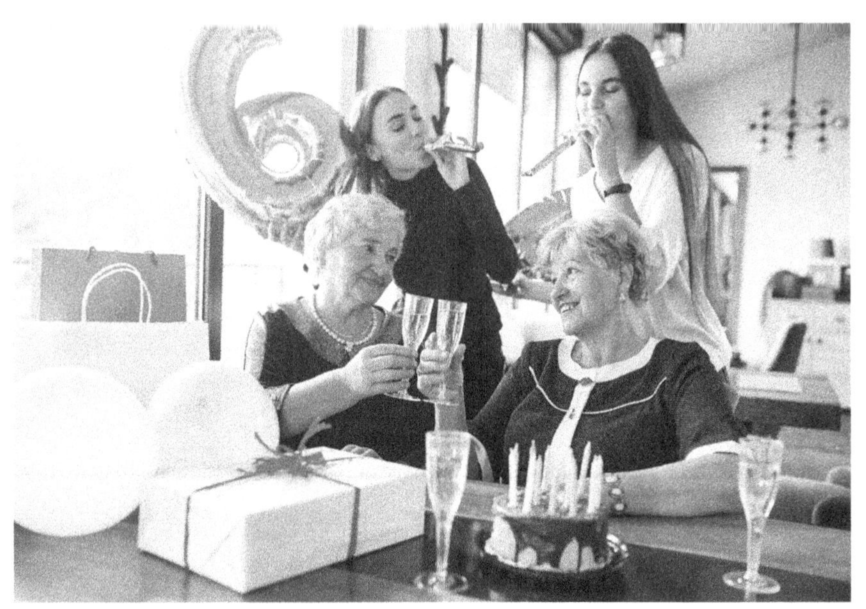

3

The Challenges of Reaching 61

"We admire people more for *trying* their hearts out than actually succeeding."

—[Sorry, I forgot.]

Getting old sucks. Sorry, but there's no other way to put it. Actually, there is: getting old doesn't have to suck. I love getting old(er) and learning new things, sharing them with others, and continuing my journey through what has been a truly fascinating and mind-blowing life.

In case you didn't know, health is the new wealth. I now have dozens of new reasons to jump outta bed and rocket myself into the day. All thanks to a choice I made a year ago: to start CrossFit.

More On Getting Old: It's Not All Bad

If you're a 20-something who just happened to pick up this book, you surely couldn't care less about what a 61 year old goes through each day. After all, you are still stinkin' gorgeous, invincible, of excellent body and mind, you stay up all night playing and partying, and wake up the next day feeling refreshed.

If you're lucky, you will someday find yourself at 61, creaky bones and all. And if you're really fortunate, your health may be pretty good, if you didn't neglect it or your wonderful mind.

For most of us, though, reaching 61 is a chore. A painful one. Our hearing loses those high notes, because the tiny hairs inside our cochlea have been sheared off by booming '70s and '80s rock and heavy metal.

The eyes suffer from elongation and thus spirit you to the optometrist once a year for new glasses. It's a small price to pay for living this long, plus you get to buy cool glasses and prescription Maui Jims or RayBans.

If you've been exposed to one of a few dozen herpes viruses, then your sense of smell takes a nosedive. As a result, your appetite is thrown way off so you compensate by eating foods and drinks with too much sugar and salt. And alcohol.

> "We have been conditioned *not* to live a full and meaningful life or make valuable contributions to society."

No, I haven't been introduced to those effin' H-viruses, but a few old friends tell me "it's the little guys that end up killing us." That's comforting.

If you've not taken proper care of the trillions of microbes in your gut, which we are only beginning to understand, then your 60s will be a painful one, perhaps even filled with diseases caused by these invisible warriors inside your gut. I discuss this more in Chapter 12.

Let's not get into how your skin, muscles, joints and bones feel. If you've not been too physically active, turning 61 will be painful and you will not wanna look in any mirror.

On the flip side, if you've been good to yourself, i.e. adopted a healthful diet, exercised regularly, stayed mentally active, enjoyed the company of family and friends, then turning 61 is a blessing.

Like I said, health is wealth, so when you reach 61, you'll see life as a miracle to respect, protect and enjoy. To top that, when you've discovered CrossFit, your whole life transforms into a world of high probabilities.

Good for you!

America Does Not Value Old People

Many years ago I talked with people in their sixties about how they lived their lives. Since they saw me as a curious sort and not some interloper, all were forthcoming with grand stories.

One woman, Amelia, told of her travels as a girl to Asia and Africa, as her father was a missionary. She spoke of living with the natives on such a deep level, and was fully integrated into their societies.

They had no idea or concept of old age. Each society was built on a system that favored young age for working, middle age for managing, and old age for sharing wisdom and looking after the grandkids.

She lamented that "America doesn't value old people, and often casts them aside to become spectators of all the shenanigans conducted by younger kids. In the old days, we observed and listened to our elders.

"They were the ones who taught us the facts of life. Not anymore. YouTube and movies and tv shows do all that."

How could she and her peers not be valued by those who haven't even lived as she had, experienced what she'd gone through?

She says, "It seems irresponsible, if not wasteful, to ignore the teachings of older folk. In American society, the stupidity of our young is celebrated in the media. YouTube features videos of abject silliness and wasted time, and our children eagerly consume it.

"Just look at the top 10 videos on YouTube on any day: absolutely *inane*. It's embarrassing to see how low our society has fallen, and what useless, empty-calorie junk our citizens are willing to accept as education and entertainment."

Why?

We Are Conditioned To Give Up Our Personal Power

Conditioning, she said. "We have been conditioned not to live a full and meaningful life or make valuable contributions to society. Leave all that to those in power or with money.

"Instead, we waste our time and effort on insignificant things that teach us nothing. Except repeat the same wasteful behaviors day in, day out. A society cannot function like that. It will waste away, its remnants a bunch of useless YouTube videos."

I was moved by her lamentation, especially when she told me how she basically dropped out of society and reinvented herself.

"If society wasn't gonna listen to me and my life wisdom, then I was gonna withdraw into a selfish life. That's when I discovered CrossFit at age 62!

"Within two years, I transformed myself into a svelte woman with fewer old-girl curves and more muscle and definition. I could hold a yoga pose for an hour, clean and jerk 125 pounds, squat 225 pounds five times, and deadlift 250 pounds. Cool!

"During those first two years, I was so preoccupied with my transformation that I forgot all about trying to fit into a society that ignored and undervalued us old girls. I found new like-minded friends to socialize with, a boyfriend who introduced me to the best sex and lovemaking ever, and a zest for life I never thought I could have.

"Like we talked about, life really is about *attitude*. How you think about things and respond to everyday stuff, something you mentioned more than once. Like you, Chris, I learned self-hypnosis from a guy who helped me quit smoking and to stop complaining about things out of my control.

"Hell, I used to love pot! Now I apply hypnosis to everything I do. It's about seeing everything with a new set of glasses and changing your perception about everything. It's also about being grateful for the things you have."

Be True To Your Own Soul

"I would like to leave some wisdom for those coming up the ladder to old age: be open to possibilities, be curious about everything but choose wisely what you engage. Everything in life is hard, so choose your 'hard.' Respect others before you dismiss them because you never know what gifts they have for you, be true to your own soul and nurture it with good food and drink and lots of exercise!

"And let's not forget my favorite: have lots of wild sex with your partner and stay in bed all day on the weekends doing it!"

There were several other poignant comments by other old folks I had planned on including here, but decided not to because Amelia touched upon the most important things to consider as we turn 61. I could've written a book based solely on her wisdom and stories. Maybe I will. As I think on it, that's not possible because Amelia is a sex goddess to her lover Ron and they are usually otherwise engaged and unavailable.

Everything considered, turning 61 has been a blessing for me, because I discovered high-intensity, intermittent exercise in the form of CrossFit. And that hour of exercise in the morning was more than enough to get me through the day, during which I also engaged in further moderate exercises to keep me off the couch.

CrossFit and Coach Pat saved my life, so there's no going back to those days of potato-couching, munching on Doritos and downing many a Dr Pepper!

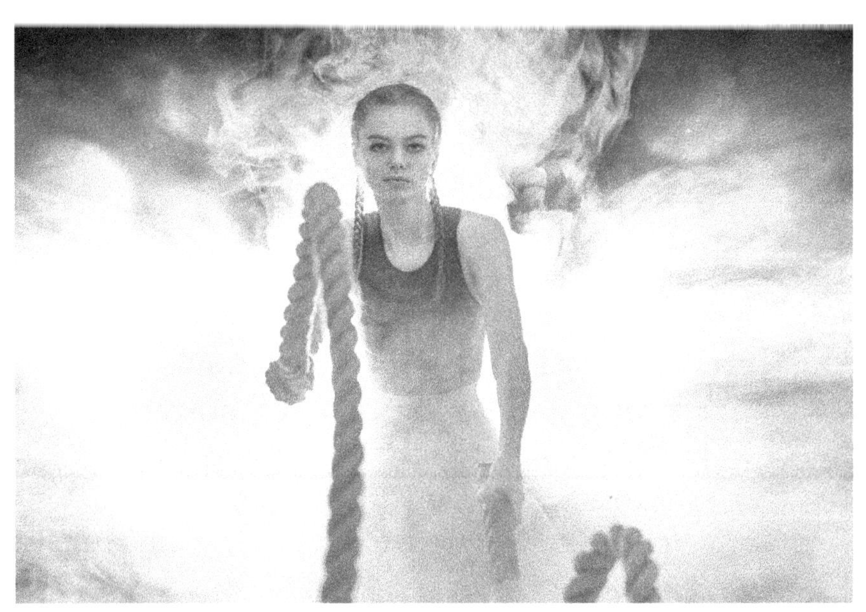

4

Smart Exercise is the Key to a Healthful Life

> "If there's ever been a hot, sweaty room filled with strong-willed, competitive, powerful, perfectionist, Type-A personalities, CrossFit would be that room."
>
> —Jessica Murden

Luckily, there've been countless medical and scientific studies that tell us exercise can cure just about everything, including a crappy disposition and saggy jowls. We are now just learning that it also positively influences our gut microbes, which in turn affect all organs and organ systems in the human body. Exercise is important!

Plus, it gives you that wonderful euphoric high from exercising at just the right pace, duration, intensity and time. What's not to love?

While it may seem an exaggeration, the fact is, being active reduces the chances of having a heart attack, getting diabetes and other metabolic and autoimmune diseases, and falling into general disrepair that will render you a potato-coucher.

This energy-rich chapter features fascinating information about the links among diet, exercise and your gut microbiome, though I do cover gut microbes and exercise in Chapter 12. When I was researching, compiling and writing it, I was captivated by all the new results from scientific and medical studies that clearly prove this important fact: we laypersons know very little about the benefits that our own gut microbes play in our everyday life.

Since I only scratch the surface of this nascent field of study, I include dozens of helpful references for you to explore. You can find them in References.

The Deceptively Simple Recipe To Good Health

Aristotle's concept of good health was simple: it was equal to *happiness*, but that virtue was completely up to the patient, not the doctor. All a doctor could do was give good, sound advice.

I love the work of innovative clinical psychologist and prolific author Dr. Nick Wignall (NickWignall.com). It is mind blowing. He has some life-changing advice for those of us who need to shake off a bad mood, for starters.

This also applies when you're anxious, depressed, stuck in a rut, and just need some kinda change for the better.

He calls it the "3 Ms":

> **1. *MOVE*.** There're boatloads of research showing that increased physical activity and exercise can have positive effects on mood. From lethargy and irritability to full-blown depression and anxiety, the mood-boosting effects of movement are powerful.
>
> The key is to realize that it doesn't take much movement to improve your mood—you certainly don't need to jog on the treadmill for an hour or pump iron 'till you're drenched in sweat.
>
> Simply getting up from your desk and going for a walk around the block can help. A few quick pushups first thing in the morning can do wonders to dispel grogginess and fatigue.
>
> And taking the kids for a walk to the park can be a quick way to de-escalate the stress and frustration of raising toddlers.
>
> The best mood booster is usually *movement*.
>
> **2. *MAKE*.** From our ancient ancestors forging arrowheads out of obsidian to the modern-day entrepreneur and mommy blogger, human beings seem wired to make stuff. And while many of us have the incredible fortune to live in a first-world country with all the luxuries and amenities that go along with it, there's a downside: We're increasingly becoming creatures

of consumption rather than creation.

We order food from GrubHub rather than making it ourselves. We hire landscapers rather than mowing our own lawns. We buy that new garbage disposal on Amazon rather than trying to fix the old one.

As we abandon our heritage as makers and creators, we're giving up one of our most powerful mechanism for feeling good—making stuff.

So the next time you find yourself in a funk, look for small opportunities to make something, fix something, or simply clean something up.

De-clutter your desk, sweep the kitchen floor, or trim the roses. Install those new electrical outlets or bake some cookies.

3. ***MEET*****.** More than our fancy problem-solving brains or our capacity for using tools and language, what sets humans apart from other species is our capacity for sophisticated relationships—for building, coordinating, and taking advantage of complex interpersonal connections.

Research shows that babies in the womb can differentiate the sound of their mother's voice, and newborns respond uniquely to other human faces. On a very fundamental level, we were born to connect.

But modern life makes it all too easy to isolate ourselves, typically under the guise of "independence." So often, the best way out of a bad mood is to simply be in the presence of someone we love. A supportive ear, an encouraging pat on the back, or a funny meme from a good friend at just the right moment can make all the difference.

We amplify our suffering when we do it alone.

When you find yourself a little down or stressed out, or upset, look for small ways to reach out and connect with someone. Pop into your coworker's office and chat for a few minutes. Send your spouse a quick "I love you" text. Call that old college buddy and catch up for 15 minutes. Sometimes even the smallest connection can make all the difference.

Get Started!

If you've been potato-couching all your life, just getting off your tush is enough to jump-start your new exercise routine. Yes, I said *potato-couching*.

It's easier to pronounce than "couch-potatoing," which is downright maddening to pronounce. It goes without saying that people who engage in potato-couching are potato-couchers. 'Nuff said there.

Former Navy SEAL, Annapolis grad, fitness instructor and author Stew Smith is one of the most creative and original workout gurus today. His workouts are legendary and they create from scratch a much better version of you.

"I used to eat garbage until I turned 50, and I was fat and miserable. I didn't actually do anything about it until I reached 60 and found CrossFit. Only then did I change my diet because the old one couldn't keep up with the demanding routines each day."

Stew tells us: "Get started by doing something easy like walking, stretching, and drinking more water than caffeine and sugar in your day.

"Seriously, just get moving by walking ten minutes before every meal, practice deep breathing while walking (box breathing) to help you relax, then stretch with some basic stretches of the legs, lower back, and arms.

"At the end of the day, you can accumulate thirty minutes or more of activity, two to three quarts of water consumed, and receive the benefits of a nice break in the middle of your day."

I love this man's work ethic, advice for all, and generally fantastic attitude. Thank you, Stew!

I could go on for pages and pages about the importance of simply *moving* as a means to good health and extending your life beyond age 61. Moving is a start to your building an exercise regimen that works specifically for you, something you can do every day or a few days a week. When you choose to move, you immediately overcome the insidious disease known as "potato-couching inertia."

Exercise Comes In Many Different Styles

These days there are so many different types of exercise for just about any kind of body type and lifestyle. There's chair yoga for senior citizens who are disabled or just not used to moving much. Extreme trail running for the, well, extreme runners in the house. Powerlifting for those who dig that kinda stuff.

Several of the women I spoke with said running is the best exercise they've ever done. They all do interval training: sprints and slow long-distance running every week. It leaves them refreshed, their skin is glowing and healthy looking, their moods are great and they sleep really well throughout the night.

They all said, too, that eating healthfully is just as important as exercising itself, because the food they put into their bodies serves as the fuel and building blocks for a strong future.

Claire M said, "I used to eat garbage until I turned 50, and I was fat and miserable. I didn't actually do anything about it until I reached 60 and found CrossFit. Only then did I change my diet because the old one couldn't keep up with the demanding routines each day. Yes, I went every day for the first year!"

And, Of Course, There's CrossFit

First conceived in 1996 and formally incorporated in 2000. Regardless of the PR, CrossFit remains the most diverse and effective exercise regimen in the world of fitness.

No other routine combines so many different exercises and combinations, although new versions of CrossFit spring up each year and attempt to avoid paying the high licensing fee to gain entrance. Some succeed because they are former crossfitters and have a large loyal following. Others just try to piggyback on the CrossFit craze.

Eric Roza saved CrossFit from a downward spiral. If it had continued under the old management, it would've crashed and made a smokin' hole. Eric's philosophy is a far cry from that of the previous owner's, but he still has not accepted the cold hard fact that most people want to exercise, not train like many crossfitters who compete in competitions and the CrossFit Games.

CrossFit Needs An Immediate Overhaul

Every single CrossFit novice I spoke with told me they hated the idea of "lifting heavy weights over my head." It was unanimous.

Plus they heard all the horror stories about people who watched videos and documentaries about elite CrossFit athletes, and wanted to be just like them. But they ended up getting hurt because they didn't train correctly. These stories have caused many to view CrossFit as a dangerous sport, one to avoid. CrossFit Headquarters and many of its affiliates are to blame for this fear.

When I started, I witnessed the elite athletes keeping to themselves and not allowing me access to their conversations because they felt I wasn't at their level.

Okay, I got that. Like one of those women I interviewed for this book said, these people (women and men) are elitists and they're unapproachable.

How do you attract new people to an atmosphere of elitism where novices are treated less than respectfully? I mean, didn't these elite athletes start somewhere, too? Like, at the bottom where I did?

Bad philosophy springs from elitism and creates an additional layer of fear in those who wish to experience this fascinating workout method. It's a large barrier to entry for us new kids.

That kind of fear has prevented thousands of people from starting CrossFit and incorporating it into their lives. I felt it, too, before I started. I just wasn't interested in doing any Olympic-style weightlifting, especially around elite athletes, plus I really effin' disliked the idea of *training*. I'm 61, for goodness' sake. I want to relax and enjoy my routines, so I now *exercise*. There's a big difference, as you now know.

I hope and pray CrossFit's new Leader, Mr. Eric Roza, is listening to this right now, because to re-launch and re-brand CrossFit as "user-friendly," he must take his tried-and-true philosophy from his days as head of Oracle Data Cloud, i.e. "relevant reach," and apply them correctly to CrossFit. In short, Mr. Roza needs to change the way people see CrossFit so it attracts a strong, loyal following of people who value exercise over training.

One Name, Two Choices

CrossFit must be divided into two different divisions, each with its own vision and purpose:

> ***CrossFit T*: worldclass *training* for athletes who wish to train hard every day so they can compete with other elite athletes at various CrossFit Opens and the Games.**
>
> ***CrossFit X*: worldclass *exercising*, a moderate routine for those of us who do not want or need intensive labor but simply wish to participate in CrossFit and become healthy, happy and fit human beings.**

Mr. Roza also needs to develop a new motto, because "forging elite fitness" is such a turn-off for me and others like me who wish to exercise and not train. I suggest that each division have its own motto or tagline.

People are frightened off by the current motto and what it represents. It's as if these elite athletes wish to keep CrossFit all to themselves and marginalize those of us who simply wanna exercise at "their" boxes.

One woman at our local box says, "Who wants to hang around a bunch of elite athletes who ignore us newbies and treat us like inexperienced children? These athletes are elitists, plain and simple, some of them even narcissists who are unapproachable.

"How can I possibly learn from someone like that? If Eric Roza is sincere about having a hundred million people doing CrossFit in ten years, then he must embrace this inescapable fact: the vast majority of those hundred million will only want to *exercise.*

"CrossFit is currently a cult that wishes to become and to be seen as an important subculture. Unfortunately, the cult was defined by the previous owner and he made it a toxic dictatorship.

"A subculture is defined by its members, many people who love and care about CrossFit and nurture it. CrossFit is far from what it wishes to be, but it's making strides in the right direction.

"My take on a new motto for exercise would go something like this: 'CrossFit: Raising a Healthy World Through Safe, Sensible Exercise and Fitness.'"

Statistics Don't Lie, Mr. Roza

Mr. Roza also needs to closely examine the statistics on CrossFit training injuries. Yes, they resemble those seen in other sports that have similar routines.

And they also tell a unique story of their own: people are getting injured unnecessarily from doing too much, too soon; overworking their body; not allowing their body to heal correctly, and thus being sidelined for a month; and performing exercises using poor techniques.

Young kids especially see pictures of elite CrossFit athletes and immediately try to become them. Doesn't work out as planned and they get injured quickly and don't return.

Current class size, in general, does not allow for adequate individual instruction on performing proper techniques. Sadly, some boxes focus on earning money and not properly training new recruits. It's a recipe for disaster.

Men are getting injured far more often than women, and the most prevalent injury involves the shoulder, primarily because of improper weightlifting and gymnastics movements. Also, men are trying to lift too much during workouts and are paying the price.

I aptly call it "dolor machista" (macho pain) and it needs to be corrected within the CrossFit community. Eric Roza, are you listening?

Statistically, women who enter CrossFit are faring better than their male counterparts and for good reason: they exercise and train more carefully and smartly, and they're more conservative in their approach to fitness, training and exercising, in general.

No, that is not a generalization. It is 100% fact. The 60-somethings will appreciate the lyrics from an old Robert Palmer song, excerpted:

But I say, it's the women today
Are smarter than the man in every way . . .
That's right, women are smarter.

Something tells me that women may be the key to evolving CrossFit into a better and safer method of working out, 'cos the guys are severely lacking now, Mr. Roza.

'Nuff said.

Two Profound Discoveries

After deciding to exercise and not train, I really dig CrossFit, especially when I put up more weight than the kids half my age.

Plus, I see a whole different me when I look in the mirror. In fact, I bought a full-length mirror and put it in a room with the most natural light.

Each morning when I rise, the first thing I do is drop down and do a long stretch, then I stand in front of that mirror and admire my handiwork.

It goes without saying that I fully embrace Olympic-style weightlifting as part of my CrossFit routine, but it did take some coaching and a lot of patience.

"Practice practice practice the tiniest of movements" became my mantra. After all, even the pros are still mastering the subtleties of their routines.

The second part of my discovery: have you ever heard of the *tabata protocol*? Tabata is a highly specific, short-duration, high-intensity interval/intermittent workout, developed in the 1990s by Japanese physiologist Dr. Izumi Tabata.

The burst exercises, when done at just the right speed, duration, intensity and rest period, burn fat and build muscle. Fast. Unlike any other kind of exercise we know of.

Strictly speaking, the 4-minute tabata protocol works in 20-second intervals of high intensity exercise, followed by 10 seconds of rest. All for a total of eight times.

The term "Tabata training" emphasizes not only the type, style and quality of the procedure or exercise itself, but also the level of intensity during the exercise that exhausts you after 7–8 sets.

Exhaustion is important because it calls into play your *anaerobic* metabolic system which, during workouts, plays a very important role in muscle building, fat loss and increased fitness.

The human body is a biological computer. We know all too well that computers can be hacked. What Dr. Tabata showed was how to hack the human computer to produce positive and beneficial results that would otherwise have eluded us during regular exercise. And it raises new questions:

What other exercise tabatas and routines can we perform to hack into our biocomputer to produce desirable effects like losing fat and increasing muscle in specific areas of the body, and strengthening tendons, ligaments and other connective tissues that support this explosive growth?

What routines can we do that will reverse diabetes and cancer, and cure what ails us?

For now, doing traditional tabatas will boost your fat metabolism quickly, especially if you do it each day or, in the case of those who cannot exercise each day, a few days a week.

It appears that burst exercises, with short rest periods, can shock your body's metabolic computer and get it to perform in novel and beneficial ways. And who knows what effects it has on our gut microbes? This is a brand-new field of study and I'm excited to be a part of it. I hope you will, too!

Blast, Burst, Flash and Shock: Biohacking Your Body

After decades of exercising, sometimes in combat conditions, I've discovered that the human body absolutely loves you when you do sudden-onset blast, burst, flash and shock exercises and movements, followed by some period of rest, mostly because you're smoked and need to recover. Also, you do not wanna injure yourself, so rest is very important.

It is abundantly clear to me that the body can be hacked into improving its baseline performance. The Tabata 20:10 routine, based on what I call the *20:10 Tabata Principle* (in honor of the 80:20 rule or Pareto Principle), is just scratching the surface of exercise "metabolic biohacking." I personally am developing a series of hourly routines anyone can do throughout the day: BlastEx. Or "blast exercises."

Every hour, you do one exercise at maximum effort for 30 seconds. I ride my Assault AirBikeElite all-out in that half-minute, then go about my routine (clean house, work on this book, grocery shopping, etc.). In the least, it gives me that shot of energy most get from coffee or an energy drink. Who knows what other benefits it provides?

Clearly, we also need a new nomenclature, the terms of which better describe these novel ideas and practices. When I use the term biohacking, I am not referring to ingesting artificial drugs, e.g. nootropics, or using enhanced gene editing. My definition refers to performing exercises and breathing to enhance your workouts and, in time, your general health and well-being.

What Dr. Tabata revealed is that to improve our performance we must engage both the aerobic and anaerobic metabolic systems at the same time during exercise. And this can be done by performing an exercise very fast, resting, then repeating this routine to exhaustion.

Dr. Tabata tells us that the maximum benefit comes when you are exhausted by the 7th or 8th set, depending on the exercise.

How? Because you have effectively used both the aerobic system in performing the exercise, and also the anaerobic system as your muscles continue the work in the absence of suitable oxygen.

Fatigue occurs when a muscle continues to contract, but does not produce the same level of force or movement. The biochemical processes during fatigue are essential to ensuring that the muscle does not perform beyond capacity and burn out. Muscle fatigue is a bioimperative that allows the muscle to rest and recover.

These are evolutionary adaptations, being able to run, jump, swim, etc. even when your muscles are out of oxygen and on the verge of seizing up or collapsing. It is fatigue that sets the upper limit of exertion, though, and prevents irreparable damage to a muscle. In short, you live to exercise smartly another day.

Putting it simply: it may just save your life if your muscles can operate effectively in the absence of oxygen for a period of time, without burning out completely.

This total engagement will increase your ability to use oxygen more efficiently as you perform any exercise, especially high-intensity work. The effect subsequently increases your endurance during exercise by using oxygen during aerobic work, and removing anaerobic byproducts, i.e. lactic acid from our muscles as quickly and efficiently as possible during the anaerobic phase, and also rapidly recycling the muscle's primary energy source: adenosine triphosphate (ATP).

When your body rewards you with the gift of a euphoric high, it's because you are performing some action or routine that's beneficial to your body.

The overall effect is increased efficiency in using oxygen and consuming ATP, and faster and more efficient recycling of anaerobic byproducts and also replenishing your ATP stores. You can perform your exercise longer, work through high-intensity exercises more efficiently, and recover faster afterward, provided you did not overwork your muscles.

Interestingly, too, biohacking can be used on specific parts of the body's muscles to produce effects only in those specific areas. It's called "site specificity" and was previously thought to be a myth.

One wonders, too, if you can lose fat in one specific area. Why wouldn't site specificity apply to fat cells? The answer remains to be discovered, though many researchers and physicians have said it is not possible. Whenever someone tells me something is not possible, I dismiss them. Anything is possible, given the right conditions.

If you wanna biohack your shoulder muscles, then you perform Tabata exercises specific to the shoulders and associated muscles: overhead press, bendover rows, etc., using a Tabata routine.

Dr. Tabata tells us more about doing shoulder work: "No effects are expected to be found in the functioning of the arm muscles. There is also specificity regarding energy-releasing systems. Anaerobic training improves the body's anaerobic capacity, whereas aerobic training elevates the aerobic capacity."

I'm excited to have found the Tabata Principle and to be putting it to work in the gym. The results I've seen in only a very short time are promising. That euphoric high is the first to appear, suggesting that some element(s) of the Tabata routine is generating that high.

When your body rewards you with the gift of a euphoric high, it's because you are performing some action or routine that's beneficial to your body. It's a positive-feedback system that benefits all, long as you do not overuse or abuse it.

Blast, burst, flash and shock exercise routines are the wave of the future, and the 20:10 Tabata strongly suggests this.

While you may not care about the science behind all this cool stuff, please understand this take-away message: even in your 60s, you can benefit greatly from Crossfit, in general, and in hacking your own biocomputer by doing Tabata routines. I strongly encourage you to experiment and develop your own "tabatas."

You will feel better almost immediately, and that effect, a long-lasting euphoric high, will become part of your new exercise routine. And if you think beyond euphoria, you will discover the importance of having muscles that can get you from point A to point B, even without needed oxygen.

A Short Intro To Your Gut Microbes and Exercise

What remains to be discovered is exactly what elements of biohacking are responsible for making us bigger, faster, stronger so we can endure exercise more efficiently. And also the specific pathways that produce that wonderful euphoric high.

A shock to your system also involves your immune system, which is usually your body's first line of defense to external stimuli and insults. Your immune system, when functioning properly, will release certain molecules and cells in response to an intense workout, which is seen by the body as an external "threat," something to act against.

In times of severe muscle and joint stress, many different compounds are produced and released into the bloodstream. Natural killer cells are among the cells called upon as part of an inflammatory response.

Some of these molecules are antioxidants that neutralize free radicals so they cannot strip electrons from beneficial and important molecules. We see this occurring in some elite athletes who overwork themselves and eventually harm their bodies.

Exercise has been shown to prevent the release or expression of many chemicals involved in the inflammatory response. Ironically, that response can be more harmful than the external stimulus or disease-causing organism itself. Yes, sometimes your body is your worst enemy. It will be interesting to study and learn how elite CrossFit athletes fare when they hit 50 and 60 years old, after having trained for many years.

The link between your gut microbes and exercise is only just being illuminated, with the first scientific research and papers being released in the past ten years. While I discuss this in detail in Chapter 12, I'd like to introduce you to some novel concepts.

The gut microbe-diet relationship has been studied more than the gut microbe-exercise connection, and is now contributing useful information we all should listen to. Exercise evokes the growth of certain gut microbes that are highly beneficial to your overall health. The time of day you exercise influences this, too, as your gut microbes have their own circadian rhythm (and other non-circadian cycles).

Example: certain bacteria that are produced more during and following exercise produce "butyrate," a bioimperative short-chain fatty acid. It is the primary energy source of cells that line the intestinal mucosa of your gut.

Who would've thought that a species of bacteria inside you would make the fuel that powers the lining of your intestines? That lining is extremely important in many ways, and when it gets leaky or tears or breaks down, we see different diseases pop up: Crohn's disease, colon cancer, consistent cramping in GI tract, persistent diarrhea, inflammatory bowel disease, gastroenteritis, etc.

It is readily apparent that these diseases are caused by lack of good bacteria and other microbes in our gut, and the proliferation of bad microbes. By potato-couching too much, eating a bad diet, and not exercising, we are destroying our own bowels and the only means of absorbing nutrients in our body.

Regular daily exercise, at least 30 minutes at a time, mediates and modulates your intestinal flora by increasing the population of good microbes and decreasing the population of bad ones. Could it be as simple as this? The short, simple answer: heck, yeah!

Exercise reduces inflammation, not only in the muscles being worked but also in your GI tract, which hosts trillions of gut microbes. Cool fact: there are more microbes in and on our body than there are our own cells, so you best start listening to what they say.

This brings up another point about your gut microbes: when the bad microbes flourish, they in turn communicate messages to your brain. They tell your brain to feed them sugar. Lots of sugar.

And I personally feel they also hack your brain into becoming a lazy, sedentary potato-coucher who lives on sugar. Results of studies and anecdotal work support this disturbing fact. And once those bad microbes take over, it is very difficult for you to ignore their orders for you to feed them more and more sugar.

In fact, to free yourself from the bonds of those nasty bad microbes, you must shock your system with a strict fast of only water for a few days, followed gradually by ingestion of dilute veggie/fruit juice, freshly prepared using a centrifugal juicer.

I've done this. It works. Thing is, you then must change your diet and maintain that adjustment in the long run.

For me, that is still a work in progress. I was raised on rich European dishes of heavy creams, butter, pasta, potatoes and well-marbled meats.

I'm sure you will do better.

So, along with regular exercise and a better diet, fasting and juicing jumpstart your GI tract to produce beneficial microbes and decrease the production of bad ones, and set you on a path to better nutrition and the production of beneficial gut microbes.

Chapter 12 features more in-depth information about your gut microbes and exercise. Since this new discipline is still in its infancy, there's not as much reliable information as I would like. Still, there's just enough to get you started on the road to re-conditioning your gut and making it work for you instead of against you.

Olympic Weightlifting: The Future Of Fitness

The misconceptions about Olympic-style weightlifting are too numerous to share here. I'll keep it simple: the various techniques and adding some weight will build your muscles, tendons, ligaments and overall physical health.

They will provide better balance and stability by building the core muscles that attach to and support your spine and the stabilizer muscles that protect and support your shoulders. Betcha you ain't heard about "stabilizer muscles," huh?

And these Olympic-style routines will also greatly increase your mobility and range of motion, which makes life a lot easier when you're 61 and beyond.

For someone who is 61, this could mean the difference between jumping out of bed in the morning or struggling to crawl out. Sure, my CrossFit sessions make me sore, but when the soreness wears off, I am left with feeling much like I did at age 27: a sense of well-being, strong, flexible, my moods are upbeat and positive. My level of enthusiasm for life has increased a lot since starting CrossFit and getting back on track to a healthy life. I've only been at it for a year, so I'm sure there're new changes in my physiology I've not yet considered. I'm still grasping the fact that I feel so much better!

And I have a higher level of endurance I didn't expect or even consider when I started exercising. This increased endurance crosses over into all aspects of my life, from carrying a 100-lb. bag of rocks to bending over many times in the garden to sitting in my suv for a long roadtrip.

My feeling is that, when enough new crossfitters discover the value of Olympic weightlifting, it will take the world by storm and become the future rage in fitness. Along with the hugely important Tabata routine and other "metabolic biohacking" exercises.

A New Definition Of *Fitness* Is Sorely Needed

If CrossFit statistics were really and truly accurate and fair, they would also include metrics like biomarkers, blood pressure, cancer markers, levels of testosterone, estrogen, progesterone, the health of your gut microbes, etc.

They would reveal the inner secrets of each athlete and measure them against all others.

Could be that there are some heart attacks waiting to happen. Or cancer. Dementia. Cardiovascular disease. Diabetes. What about drug abuse? Coke. Marijuana. Performance-enhancing drugs.

If some great athlete has diabetes and takes insulin, or they use marijuana, are they still considered "fit"?

What about mental health? If they suffer from anxiety and depression, are they still fit? What if they take anti-anxiety medication? Are they still fit?

Are they, their lifestyle, morals, standards, etc. a model for others to emulate and follow? If they're outside the norm, are they still fit?

After considering every possible biometric, physical and mental and spiritual, social and psychological, we then would have a new measure of "fitness."

Beyond that, who then decides what *fitness* truly is?

Ask me? I say it is up to each of us, because our body is different from the next person's. I am a fit 61-year-old man, but I cannot perform a 300-lb. clean and jerk. Nor is my level of testosterone that of a 20-year-old man. I can run on a treadmill, but not on asphalt.

So what?

I feel great, have a wonderful attitude, do positive things for myself and others, am productive every day, and go to bed knowing I am a good person who does his job well and also does good in this world.

Could I be "fitter"?

Of course. Question is, how much more time, effort, energy and money am I willing to give to be just a bit more fit? There are upper limits, or maxima, I place on all variables like time and energy. I am willing to do what it takes to meet my goals, and I will not go beyond that. Same goes for you: find your *happy maxima* for fitness.

CrossFit: A Combination Of Many Good Things

There is no one key to extending your beautiful life. It is, as Aristotle taught us, a combination of many different and important ingredients that act in harmony to produce not only good health but happiness, as well.

About the quote at the beginning of this chapter: please do *not* be scared off, thinking CrossFit is filled only with Type-A personalities. Far from it. Example: I'm a quiet, shy, Type-Z introvert who loves being alone, working alone, hiking alone, eating alone, watching Ted Lasso alone, and traveling alone.

And I love CrossFit like I love breathing, perhaps even more than those Type-As! I feed off the energy of my fellow crossfitters, and give back the same to them, hence, my Type-Z character.

There are many different personality types among those who wish to exercise and not train. In fact, those who choose exercising probably represent much more diverse personality types.

It's your choice whom you interact with.

The ones I've met and exercise with are wonderful human beings.

A gentle reminder: *potato-couch and potato-couching* have just been added to the English lexicon. You're free to add *potato-coucher*.

potato·couch | pəˈtādō,ˈkouCH |
verb
Sit for hours and days on a couch, while watching endless movies, tv shows and other forms of entertainment, consuming thousands of calories of delicious junk food, soft drinks, beer, wine, marijuana, etc., and contributing to an early demise.
Also *potato-couching* and *potato-coucher*.

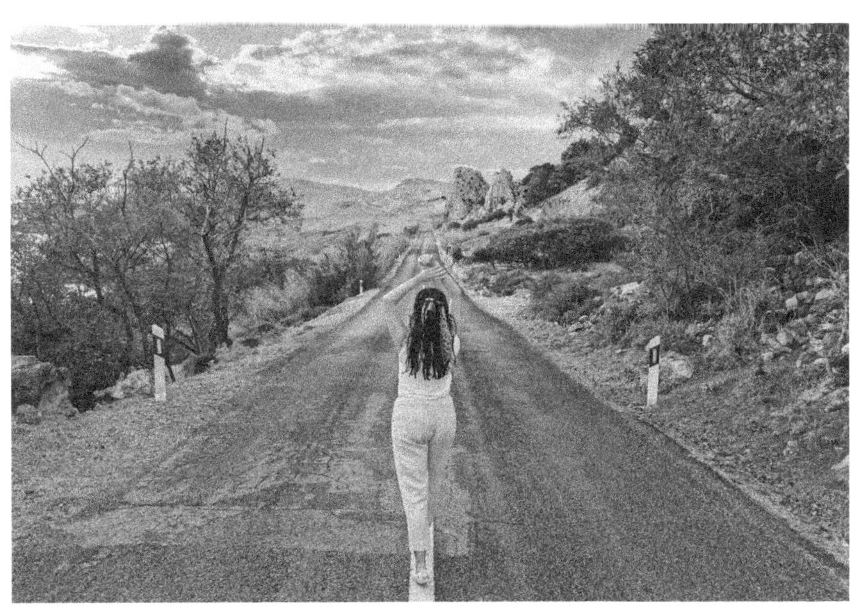

5

A 27-Step Program for Starting CrossFit

"Decide your own path, you will."
—Yoda

Before you set foot in a CrossFit box, get a thorough physical exam from your primary-care physician, including range-of-motion test, flexibility test and overall mobility test. Have them do a complete blood workup and urinalysis.

Also request they test your hormone levels (e.g. testosterone, estrogen, progesterone, etc.), thyroid function, liver panel, vitamin B12 and D3 levels, insulin and blood glucose levels, hemoglobin A1c.

Though very new, get a test of your gut microbes to see if they're out of balance. Your gut bacteria, yeasts and other fungi, viruses and miscellaneous microbes all form a complex ecosystem that influences every organ and organ system in your body, so it's important to learn about its composition and to keep it happy. I discuss this more in Chapter 12.

It might also be beneficial to see a chiropractor for an exam and maybe even an adjustment. I see one once a year and he's great at looking at my spine and doing minor corrections so everything functions well.

Chiropractors come in all shapes and styles. Some will charge you an arm and a leg for an x-ray or scan of your spine. Ask for a discount. A good chiropractor will give you excellent advice and guidance about how best to exercise your body in its current state.

The chiropractor evaluates your gait, motion and posture, looks for and identifies anything that may be restricting your movements and performance, carefully examines the soft tissues (muscles, tendons, ligaments, nerves and nerve sheaths, fascia and other connective tissue that may be restricting movement, and works the affected area(s) to restore full function.

Though I suggest doing these tests to get a good baseline of your current fitness, please do not *overprepare*. That would be a sign of avoidance, fear and procrastination. Who wants to open up *that* can o' worms?

Just dive in.

The Results Of An InBody Test Will Shock You!

Some places including CrossFit boxes also have a cool InBody machine that you stand on, with your hands gripping two electrodes. From the InBody website: "What does your weight really represent? When you step on a scale, you can't see how much muscle or fat you have. All you see is how heavy you weigh.

"Go beyond the scale with the InBody Test, a non-invasive body composition analysis that provides a detailed breakdown of your weight in terms of muscle, fat, and water on an InBody Result Sheet.

"An InBody Test can take anywhere from 15-120 seconds, depending on the model used . . . When you measure your weight, what are you actually seeing?

"Weight alone is a poor indicator of health because it does not distinguish fat from muscle. The InBody divides your weight into water, muscle, and fat.

"How much muscle do you have in your arms? Your legs? With the InBody Test, discover how many pounds of lean mass you have distributed in each portion of your body. See which exercises bring out the best results and get balanced gains.

"BMI is an inaccurate way of measuring how healthy you are.

Instead, focus on your body fat to weight ratio, also known as Percent Body Fat. Measuring your Percent Body Fat allows you to better your health from the inside out so you focus on fat loss and not just weight loss.

"Knowing how much fat and muscle you have is only the beginning. With your baseline set, continuously taking the InBody Test allows you to monitor and track the changes in your body."

Even more important is the fat-to-muscle ratio (F:M). It should be relatively low. Too much fat, especially in the midsection, can lead to dysbiosis (imbalance of gut bacteria) that in turn can cause many other preventable diseases and ailments.

I do the test every two months to measure my exercise and fitness progress. Biofeedback like this is priceless.

To find an InBody location near you, go to this link:

https://inbodyusa.com/support/nearest-testing-location/

The overall biomarkers of these blood, urine and InBody tests will give you a good baseline of your current health.

This Ain't Yo' Mama's Betty Crocker Recipe For Fudge Brownies

1. First, commit 100% to making a significant change in your life. Write down all the pros and cons for exercising and feeling better.

Once you've convinced yourself this is for you, search online for CrossFit boxes near you. If you can visit more than one, that's even better. Then decide how far you are willing to drive to exercise.

I'm lucky: my box is less than 10 minutes away from my home. When I first contacted a box, long before I found my current one, I was usherd into their Bootcamp program, which has some high-intensity workouts but with no weights, i.e. barbells and dumb bells.

I did this consistently for about 6 months and, to be honest, didn't get much out of it. Sure, it depends what you put into it. But I needed the high-intensity workouts and weightlifting that CrossFit offered.

So I looked around for a new box. Soon as I started learning the CrossFit routines, I was hooked. In just a few months I was seeing dramatic changes in my level of energy, mood, muscle mass and tone, body chemistry, etc.

So, I highly recommend your *not* doing Bootcamp and just starting CrossFit. The benefits will astound you.

2. Research reviews about each box, ask around to see if anyone knows the reputation of the box(es). Pay particular attention to negative reviews. Even the disgruntled person who lasted only a week may have something important and useful to offer in their review.

After I read reviews, I just walked into the first box I exercised at for a few months, and talked with the head coaches. The owner was cold and distant and couldn't give a hoot about me. That turned me off.

By visiting both boxes, I was able to sense their vibe. The first one was not good. The second was my slice of heaven, and it's where I still exercise today. Please be patient when choosing a suitable CrossFit box for you. It's kinda like choosing a life partner or a home, so do your due diligence before committing.

3. Call and make an appointment to meet in person with the head trainer, or at least with one of the advanced trainers. I've talked with many CrossFit coaches and found just about all of them knowledgable enough to field questions.

You can tell who is a good coach and teacher and who isn't by their level of patience and interest when you ask questions. You are looking for a good strong personality, patient demeanor, and one who is knowledgeable about the exercise routines and techniques.

Steer clear of those "used-car salesmen" who try to sell you all their nutritional supplements and drinks, their shiny equipment, etc.

4. Please dress in appropriate workout attire when you meet the coach. Ask the instructors at each box what's appropriate before you go. They may ask you to perform a few exercises to test your level of fitness, flexibility and overall range of motion and movement. I've found yoga pants or soft, flexible workout pants or shorts are best.

Wear comfortable workout shoes or runners if you haven't already invested in a dedicated CrossFit shoe. Thickness and style of socks is up to you. I started out wearing heavy Thorlo socks (low cut for running), but later switched to very thin ones, which I now prefer.

Thicker socks allow too much movement inside the shoe, and this is not good when you're doing heavy lifting like squats where the feet must be well planted, or when you're doing quick side-to-side movements.

5. Ensure the box has hours that meet your schedule. If you're a morning person, then ensure you get to exercise before noon. Night owls need evening sessions. If they cannot accommodate your needs, make a request for extended or different hours. No luck? Try another CrossFit box.

If there's not another one near you, consider doing private sessions with a seasoned CrossFit instructor at times that suit you and your schedule.

One of the most important things about exercise is doing it at the right time for you, i.e. when you body is ready for it. The flip side is to exercise at odd times so your muscles and body get used to different times and schedules. The upside is that your body can react well to stress at all times, not just at 9 am or 5 pm. Remember: while you may prefer a routine, your body has a mind of its own and it likes to be shocked from time to time.

6. Regardless of the rates, ask for a monthly discount: senior, first-responders, military, veteran, etc. Always ask for discounts! I pay less than most others because I asked for special rates for regular CrossFit and private sessions.

If possible, strike up a chat with the owner of the box. If they are not accessible, then try the senior-most coach or instructor. Develop a rapport with them, ask them poignant questions, get a little personal with details about your motives and motivation for starting CrossFit. Ask for their advice.

When you've built even a small relationship with them, you can then make the Big Ask:

"May I please have a discount on your rates? I am willing to pay up front for six months, or even a year to receive your generous new rate." If you don't ask you pro'ly will not get what you want and need.

7. Ask about private sessions with a seasoned coach. If you're more comfortable with a female, ask for one. I suggest doing 30-minute sessions, because they are more concentrated than regular classes and focus on specific muscle groups with exercises that will drain your energy in no time.

I'm smoked at the end of my privates sessions, and I get so much more out of them than regular CrossFit sessions, which are sometimes too noisy and distracting to me. Don't get me wrong, I love blastin' music most of the time, but not when I'm trying to concentrate on doing a 375-lb. squat correctly.

You might also prefer one-on-one private classes because they're much less noisy than regular classes. Plus, there're no other students to distract you or your coach.

Again, ask for a discount, using the simple method I suggest in #6.

8. Ask how the box works with inexperienced people, especially seniors. Do they have a specific workout routine, or do they simply place newcomers in regular classes and show them the exercises and proper techniques as you go along?

I've found that most boxes will try to put newcomers in their Bootcamp sessions. Don't do it.

Talk with the owner or a senior coach about starting you off in regular CrossFit classes. Tell them you know the value of incorporating Olympic-style weightlifting and other routines with weights, and you want to do them and learn proper techniques. And no, you do not want to start off in Bootcamp!

9. I say this again! Request *not* to be placed in a Bootcamp, which does not incorporate weightlifting. I found it to be a waste of time for me and a good money-maker for the box, especially for females and older folks. I recommend jumping right into CrossFit and learning the techniques as you progress, as stated in #8.

You must be firm in your conviction not to do Bootcamp. I've seen CrossFit coaches being schooled by their owners on how best to get as many people into Bootcamp as possible. Their goal is to make money, then push the best of their students into CrossFit later on.

10. More on private lessons: do take private lessons and ask to learn all the exercises and techniques. Thirty minutes, once a week is a good start. To supplement those, I also recommend going to at least two CrossFit classes each week.

If this proves to be too much for you, then do the private session and only one regular CrossFit class until you work up the stamina and endurance.

In time, say, about six months, you will be able to do two privates each week, plus at least two regular CrossFit sessions. In your privates, you will further develop all the weightlifting techniques, so you can perform them correctly and safely in CrossFit sessions.

Without proper instruction in Olympic weightlifting, you could pull muscles and injure joints.

11. Do not be afraid to ask anyone a question about how to improve your performance, technique, or even diet and nutrition. Most people I've encountered are very friendly and knowledgeable, and are eager to assist a newcomer. CrossFit exercises require specific techniques and movements. They also require that you eat the right foods and drink the right fluids.

Some have wiggle room, others do not. As a senior, you need to be careful not to injure yourself before you begin this new exercise routine. Have your coach take you aside and show you proper techniques.

Our box has one outstanding nutritionist who coaches me on how to change my bad eating habits. I'm moving along slowly. But surely.

You will only discover them if you interact with people, ask questions, and share your personal goals. Plus, socializing is good for the heart, mind and soul.

12. Watch those experienced crossfitters who have good techniques, and adopt them. Go to other Crossfit classes and observe. If possible, go to CrossFit-sanctioned events and games. The pros make it all look easy, because they have excellent techniques. Local boxes also have amateur events for teens, adults and seniors. To me, they're more fun than watching the CrossFit Games!

When you watch an expert perform an exercise, you are learning how to do it yourself. It's just a different form of learning. When you are alone, close your eyes and "image" those same movements a pro did, but imagine you are the one doing it.

It's called "imaging" and it's a very effective training technique and form of meditation. When you go to bed, tell yourself to dream about a particular technique you wish to learn or improve. It may take some time, but your subconscious will comply with your wishes and begin to perform those exercise techniques, with you at the steering wheel. Again, very effective learning technique, and all it takes is your seeding the information into your subconscious at bedtime.

Ask more questions! Take videos of those who have good techniques. Study those videos at home. Talk them over with your coach and then perform in front of them. Get feedback on your own movements so you can improve on the spot.

13. At home or work, watch Instagram and YouTube videos by seasoned CrossFit pros and keely observe and study their techniques. Practice on your own and with your coach.

Continually observing those who have excellent techniques will allow you to improve even when you're not in a class or private session. Yes, it bears repeating!

I highly recommend watching Instagram videos by ShenZhen Weightlifting (@shenzhenweightlifting). These guys employ the same method of training as sushi schools, they spend the first year or two learning how to make the perfect cup of rice. In ShenZhen, they spend many months on each individual movement of each barbell exercise until they perfect it.

Essentially, they take a barbell exercise and break it down to its most basic elements, and have each student do just one movement at a time, over and over, until the student becomes proficient. Then they are permitted to add the next movement in the series.

Their method of training should be taught here in the US.

Unfortunately, as one CrossFit instructor told me, ironically, most people aren't willing to take the time, spend the money, or have the patience to train at that basic level, even though it's the smartest and safest method in the world.

14. Each day, renew your commitment to continuing your CrossFit routines. If necessary, talk with your coaches about your state of mind, and let them assuage any fears or misconceptions you may have. Attitude is everything. Keep yours in top shape.

No one teaches us how to maintain a healthy mind. Our thoughts are largely shaped when we are children, and sometimes when we are stressed we revert back to the behavior of a 10 year old.

Find a good role model to assist you in developing a good, strong way of thinking and dealing with stress and the associated anxiety we often feel.

CrossFit can chemically alleviate the negative feelings caused by stress, but it cannot show you how to deal with stress. My favorite go-to mental-health profession is a seasoned Licensed Clinical Social Worker (LCSW). It's worth the $100 an hour you will spend to have her put your head on correctly.

You don't have to see her every week. Maybe a few times a year. More at first to get that initial adjustment, then less often. My LCSW gave me great mental exercises to do for the first few months I saw her.

After a few helpful sessions, I felt great and so I discontinued my sessions with her.

15. WARNING: Be very patient with your progress each day, week and month, as it will take at least *six* months for you to see any real positive effects and improvement in your routines and exercises.

It took me just over six months, and when it came I was super-jazzed. My muscle definition in my shoulders appeared first, then mild weight loss, better definition in my legs then arms, thicker muscles in legs, increased strength in all muscles, greater flexibility when doing all exercises, plus I just felt much better!

I was always patient. For me, the journey is more important than the destination. Sadly, reaching the destination is often anticlimactic.

You must understand the difference between pain and injury. Talk it over with your CrossFit coach. Pain can be mild muscle tears after a strenuous workout. Or it can be painful exhaustion after a tabata. Injury is when you seriously tear or pull a muscle, tendon or ligament, and the injury requires considerable time to heal and rehabilitate.

Please do not quit just because you feel pain during or after your workouts. If it's not an injury, then press on. The pain from working out shall pass.

You will learn about "delayed-onset muscle soreness," which is thought to be caused by small muscle tears as you over-work your muscles. To grow, they just be broken down to some extent. Or so researchers and medical professionals tell us.

My personal knowledge and experience: exercise evokes many different chemical reactions and cascades. In turn those produce other reactions and release other chemicals in various cells, tissues and organs of our body. Some respond to inflammation when muscles tear. This very reaction can cause pain.

Others are involved in muscle, tendon, ligament and connective-tissue repair and localized replacement. Ibuprofen and stretching, especially using foam rollers, can assuage the pain and help promote faster healing.

Pain appears to accompany the building and stabilizing of muscle, joints and bones. It is an integral part of the growing process when we exercise our body above and beyond normal daily movements.

Most people fear pain so they try to avoid it. Without pain, though, there is no growth. We must learn to appreciate and respect this fact.

My coach says, "Embrace the pain so you can embrace the journey."

16. If you have an unhealthful diet, see a nutritionist about changing it. Stay away from alcohol, cigarettes (and/or cigars), illegal drugs, etc. Some people swear by the therapeutic effects of marijuana. It works for some people, not others. I found that you have to consume a lot of it to get any beneficial therapeutic affect. Sure, you may produce some helpful effects, but you'll be stoned the whole time.

About diet and nutrition: I recommend changing your diet slowly.

Try removing something harmful from your diet for one week a month. Then after three months, do two weeks. Every three months, remove more garbage until it's gone from your new diet.

I suggest every three months because it takes the human body that long to respond to changes in chemistry, e.g. when you start taking a new drug or supplement.

There are of course some exceptions: alcohol has an almost immediate effect, producing a "buzz." Opium and its derivatives produce instant euphoria.

Not that you'll ever smoke it, but crack immediately hijacks the brain's dopamine transport system, forcing dopamine to persist within the synapse of dopamine-releasing neurons.

Since dopamine is one of the neurotransmitters involved in the normal pleasure and reward system that keeps us coming back to CrossFit, because, along with other molecules, it produces euphoria and an unusual "high."

Your brain's mesolimbic dopamine system is involved in pleasure and reward, and emotions and motivation. It is stimulated by many different reinforcing actions and behaviors: food, sex, CrossFit, and illegal drugs including cocaine.

When you take illegal drugs, too much dopamine collects in the synapse to produce an artificial "high," an unnatural euphoria that is amplified, making you feel very uncomfortable. Enough about illegal drugs. Just know any high you get from taking them is short lived and could lead to disastrous effects.

Illegal drugs and CrossFit do not mix so don't go there, please.

As I stated in #11, don't be afraid to ask questions, especially about diet and nutrition. You may have to pay for professional advice and counseling, but it is well worth the investment in your good health and well-being.

17. Drink at least one gallon of water each day, no exceptions. Staying hydrated is the single biggest step you take each day. Being dehydrated causes all cells in your body, including muscles and neurons, to lose molecular water.

One example: when the concentration of water decreases, the

apparent or relative concentration of solutes that are soluble in water *increase* and can have unpleasant consequences until you re-hydrate again.

In muscles, the concentration of calcium goes up, causing severe muscle cramps. In the GI tract, the same happens. When magnesium levels increase, the effect causes muscle cramping and diarrhea, not to mention light-headedness and vertigo, among other deleterious effects.

Think about when you drink a bottle of magnesium sulfate to loosen the fecal matter in your intestines. It has a high concentration of magnesium. Very effective. Also very painful in high concentration. Stay hydrated to avoid causing your electrolytes to shift out of balance. It throws off your body's chemical and metabolic equilibrium.

18. Get plenty of quality sleep. For some, this is eight hours. Others, maybe six or nine. Only you know how well you sleep. Avoiding alcohol at night is a good practice. Same with cigarettes.

Sleep is important, especially deep sleep. When you go into a deep state of sleep, yoour body undergoes major repairs on so many levels, including fixing and rebuilding DNA within your genes; repairing damaged muscles, tendons, ligaments, bones and soft connective tissue.

You also dream, which is how the body's subconscious mind communicates with both you and the spirit entities outside our body. Dreams and dreaming are an important way for your subconscious to tell your body what it needs, e.g. exercise more!

It's that little voice in the back of your head, nagging at you to do something important. Actually, it's much more complex than that, but that's for another book.

19. Learn the art of stretching and yoga. Yoga sessions do not always incorporate proper stretches for CrossFit exercises, but yoga complements other stretching exercises very well. Your CrossFit coaches will school you on proper stretching techniques. Some CrossFit boxes even have yoga classes, so please take advantage of them.

Stretching is most important because, during CrossFit workouts, muscles and connective tissues that bind and protect muscles contract a lot and sometimes at high frequency. CrossFit exercises sometimes cause muscles to remain contracted slightly after the workout. It produces that uncomfortable feeling of tightness.

It is not a good idea to allow your muscles to remain tight, as you can easily pull them and cause painful injury that will take weeks to heal.

The only safe way to tease apart these contracted muscles is to artificially pull them apart by stretching and yoga. There are many different types and styles of stretches, so please consult your CrossFit and yoga instructors.

There is a wonderful supplement to stretching and yoga: soaking in a hot magnesium sulfate (epsom salt) bath will cause magnesium (and sulfates) to diffuse across your skin. Magnesium is important for muscle growth and maintenance, so your body will welcome this boost in healing.

Don't worry: your body tightly regulates the concentration of magnesium (and other substances) in your blood, so when it reaches optimum levels, your body routes it to the kidneys where it is harmlessly excreted in urine.

Those who take regular epsom salt baths report feeling much more relaxed and less painful after a workout, whether it's CrossFit or some other routine. So if you're not concerned about a high water bill, take regular magnesium baths.

20. Get outside in nature and have fun! Go out on the town and socialize with other people! Forming bonds with others will lift your mood, something positive you take with you to your CrossFit sessions. When you step outside and hyperjump to warp speed, you outrun your own shadow.

Remember: attitude is everything. Having great neurochemistry and general chemistry is like having $100 million dollars in your bank account. Yes, really. It's worth more, in fact.

Everything you see, hear, touch at any time affects your mood and how your nervous, endocrine, and immune systems react and function.

Your current working or living environment can produce anxiety, depression and a feeling of helplessness. These issues increase your blood pressure, heart rate, and create deleterious issues in other body organs and systems. Combined, they also suppress your immune system, thus giving way to illness, disease and, if prolonged, even death.

Getting out in nature can erase all those issues, but it takes time, i.e. taking walks or hikes each day or week, as long as you are consistent. When you are one with nature, you suddenly feel at ease and calm. Our genetic makeup has blessed us with the ability to sense the beauty of nature.

Get out in nature, get connected, absorb the wonderful atmosphere, and then take those feelings back home with you. The effects we feel from nature last long after we depart and return to our concrete jungle.

21. Read books! It will keep your mind in good working order and teach you some stuff in the process. While you're at it, read about all the cool things people have written about exercise, food and nutrition, sleep, etc.

Our brain is programmed to receive valuable information, so put it to use by reading a good book each day. Doing so stimulates certain neural pathways and synapses in the brain, and forms new connections.

Some of these connections later become "hardwired" and are stored in our multiple memory banks.

We've seen the ill effects of not using your beautiful mind: gradual wasting away, loss of social skills, decreased levels of interest in life, anxiety, depression, dementia, etc.

Reading isn't just fundamental, it's a vital part of a healthful life.

22. Have a hobby or two, like writing. Yes, writing. How does this assist you in CrossFit? Indirectly, it helps you focus on something other than exercise, and trains your mind to stick to something from start to finish.

It is good for the soul because it is a labor of love. All that pours into your general reservoir of energy you need for CrossFit.

Like reading books, writing something as small as a list of wishes or dreams boosts your mood, reduces general anxiety, prevents the onset of depression, lowers blood pressure and heart rate (unless your hobby is doing 100-meter sprints).

23. Teach someone something. It will prepare you to instruct yourself in CrossFit and to become your own mentor when no one else is around to assist you. Teaching a subject also trains your brain to develop new synaptic connections in areas involved in learning and memory, especially the hippocampus.

My hypothesis about this: those new neural circuits you develop from teaching can also influence how you learn CrossFit exercises from someone who teaches you.

Showing another human being how to do something or perform some action is also good for the heart and soul. Your feeling of well-being is boosted because we are genetically programmed to be social and helpful, to assist our fellow human beings.

That great euphoric feeling we get is our reward for coming to someone's aid. It is a self-reinforcing cycle that keeps you coming back for more.

24. We are also programmed to show gratitude and to be thankful for the things we are and have. Be grateful for everything you have and are. Show gratitude. Give unselfishly. Without expecting anything in return.

When we do so, we acknowledge all the positive things in our life, and cease to take anything for granted. Gratitude helps you feel more good strong emotions, appreciate good experiences, improve health, handle difficult situations better, and you also build stronger relationships with those around you.

It's no surprise that praying and generally giving thanks improves our mood, and thus it changes our neurochemistry for the better. You don't have to be religious or even spiritual. Just take a quiet moment to say thank you, even if you're talking to the sky or a tree.

We can express thanks and gratitude for things in our past, present and future.

Our past: growing up in a healthy environment and learning cool lessons, meeting great people, being mentored by someone special.

Our present: the family, friends and colleagues we have, our good job, money to feed, clothe and shelter us.

Our future: remaining positive and optimistic about our life and all in it.

When we show gratitude, we experience an immediate sensation of social-induced euphoria, though to a lesser extent than the exercise-induced high from doing CrossFit or some other form of high-intensity exercise or work.

25. Laugh. They tell us that laughter is the best medicine and they're right. It's been proven over and over again that laughter can improve your mood, even when you're depressed and anxious.

The physical benefits of laughter and humor: improves and increases your immune system and its responses to harmful stimuli that enter your body, decreases the stress hormone cortisol, relaxes tight muscles, increases your response to pain and allows you to cope better, prevents cardiovascular disease, etc.

The mental health benefits: increases happiness and joy, lifts your general mood, decreases stress and improves your response to it, helps you bounce back from difficult situations better, etc.

Social benefits are numerous, too, even if you're not too social or sociable: forges new friendships and relationships, even with strangers, magnetically attracts good people to you, brings good people together as a team and produces positive results in work and play, builds stronger bonds among members of a team or group, etc.

26. Breathe! Learn how to breathe correctly, especially to reduce stress and anxiety. My colleague Navy SEAL Stew Smith has some great breathing exercises for you. His information is in the References chapter.

Briefly, you can use this simple deep-breathing technique to calm yourself down in less than a minute: 1. Deep inhalation for 4 seconds. 2. Hold your breath for 5 seconds. 3. Blow out the breath slightly forcefully, pursing your lips, for 6 seconds. Repeat this 10 times. Feels great, doesn't it? You can do this anytime, anywhere. Best of all, you can repeat it as often as you wish.

Using a good, deliberate breathing technique has been proven to positively affect all major organs and systems in the human body. Research results show us that you can perform a breathing exercise for just a few minutes and get immediate results, simply by hacking your vagus nerve.

Besides alcohol and some drugs, deep breathing is the fastest way to take control of your body and change something for the better. A deep-breathing exercise can produce results in mere seconds. If you're stressed, with feelings of anxiety, your deep-breathing exercise can reduce it or make it disappear altogether.

Indian yoga practitioners have been doing deep-breathing work for centuries, and have documented the benefits, some of which I've listed above.

Your body's normal stress response has been programmed to be beneficial, believe it or not. In times of stress, the heart rate and blood pressure go up considerably to respond to a particular stimulus. It may be someone trying to harm you, so your body prepares to defend you, if not go on the attack.

Unfortunately, our modern world has created thousands of stressful stimuli that impinge on us every day, and this stress artificially elevates our stress level. We respond by fighting, fleeing, freeing up, flipping out like a crazy person, or attemting to fraternize with the "enemy" or the nasty stimulus that attempted to harm us.

Even in the throes of combat, you can control your breathing. First, you must notice that your breathing is artificially elevated. Then you talk to yourself to calm down your responses.

Then you employ your secret weapon: deep-breathing work. It will almost immediately calm you down, which then allows you to think more clearly.

Face it, breathing correctly has its benefits.

27. Smile! Like laughter, a smile causes certain muscles of the face and neck to contract, thus stimulating cranial nerve VII, or the facial nerve. Its axonal branches innervate all the muscles of expression around the eyes and mouth.

When we smile, it produces a feeling of well-being. To me, happiness is something else entirely: a product or side effect of productive movement and accomplishment, and is different from a feeling of well-being.

Smiling shares all the physical, mental and social benefits of laughter, and also has some unique traits of its own. A smile can be seen. Laughter can be heard. Combined, the results are wonderful!

People love to see another person smile. You are naturally drawn to them and want to meet and interact with them. A person who smiles is seen as more attractive, even beautiful.

Those who see you smile often find you more successful, so they want to be around you and share in your success, if even vicariously.

Smiling is seen as the fountain of youth: when others see you smile, they find that you look and act younger. I personally have found that smiling puts people at ease. I disarm even the toughest of men with a simple smile. They then know I am not a threat to them. Back in the day, I bought them many a beer or Jack Daniels.

The sight of a smile in public also suggests success, because that person appears confident, happy and positive. They must do well in life with all that enthusiasm.

How Most People Fail When Starting CrossFit

Face it, some people are born to fail for so many reasons. They can't help it. Failure follows them everywhere. Thank goodness, this is not you or what defines your life story.

Disappointments arise primarily from two main reasons in life: 1. Unexpressed communications, i.e. not sharing what's on your mind, especially with yourself; and 2. Unfulfilled expectations, i.e. unrealistic assumptions about success are not met.

People largely fail to commit to CrossFit because they have not set realistic goals. And this happens because they have not discussed the possibilities and probabilities of their own success in doing CrossFit.

People who start CrossFit usually do not have realistic expectations, so when those expectations are not met, they quit.

They also fail because they don't tolerate the pain that comes with muscle building, joint enhancing, bone stabilizing, flexibility improvement, etc.

Remember Westley, aka Dread Pirate Roberts, in *The Princess Bride*? He tells the princess, "Life is Pain. Anyone who says different is trying to sell you something."

Good point, his.

The fact is, anytime we grow, pain ensues. Get used to it. As my Coach says, "Embrace the pain, embrace the journey." There, I said it twice.

Yup, most people who quit CrossFit after only a few months should have read this book before starting. I was there where they were. I felt pretty much the same kinda pain they did. I learned long ago that pain is a good part of life.

If you don't like pain, then change the way you look at it, how you react and respond to it. Me? I taught myself to see pain as an orgasmic moment. I don't hafta tell you how that changed my life. And no, I'm not addicted to pain.

If you're thinking of quitting CrossFit before you see some positive results, discuss your expectations with your instructor or coach. They will encourage you to relax and be patient. I've already stated that it takes about six months for you to see any real progress in CrossFit.

So why not just enjoy the journey, have multiple orgasms like I do along the way, and just have fun? Six months ain't nothin'.

The good news about enduring and persevering is that when you overcome a very difficult event, act, or situation, you come out the other side much stronger than before. And you now have new-found knowledge about yourself: you can take the pain and still succeed.

I'm not simply telling you to take the pain without context. Again, pain is part of the process of growing, so please see it that way, accept it, and get on with your beautiful life in CrossFit.

The other main reason people fail is not their own fault. Their body is not prepared physically, mentally, chemically to do CrossFit. As we get older, we tend to neglect our body and so it falls into disrepair.

I told you earlier in this chapter that you needed to see your primary-care physician and a chiropractor to get a baseline foundation of your body's health and your fitness.

You also need to check your body's level of *magnesium*, epsecially if you're diabetic and/or drink too much alcohol. Low concentrations of magnesium lead to lethargy, tiredness, low energy, weakness, muscle cramps and loss of appetite. I mention magnesium deficiency because most people have low levels and don't even know it.

CrossFit: Just Do It, Would You Please?

Please consider my 27 suggestions about how to start enjoying CrossFit, and also my statements about working through the pain and succeeding. Once again, please do not *overprepare*. Just dive in!

If you choose to exercise and not train, then you will start off easy and work your way up to a comfortable level of workout routines each week. In time, you will see improvement in all you do. Again, please be patient.

Honestly, there is no easy way to start, so establish a good sound routine from the beginning and set yourself up for success, keeping in mind that you may not see any positive changes for six months.

Nothing good in life is easy. Anything truly worth your time, effort, money and passion has a price, sometimes steep. Sacrifices must be made in the spirit of reaching your goals.

There will be cries and tears. That's okay! Crying releases special stress hormones from the body. Afterward, you feel calm, relaxed, with lower blood pressure and anxiety. Go ahead and cry a jag! It's part of your CrossFit journey.

You must be willing to work hard and be consistent about it to *earn* your new health and fitness. Nothing is easy, but I promise you that, after six months, you will see marked improvement in your health, fitness and well-being.

The CrossFit community is 100% committed to ensuring your success, first starting on your journey and then continuing well into the future. Like many other things in life and CrossFit, it is a self-reinforcing cycle of goodness.

Whatcha waitin' for, *Christmas*!?

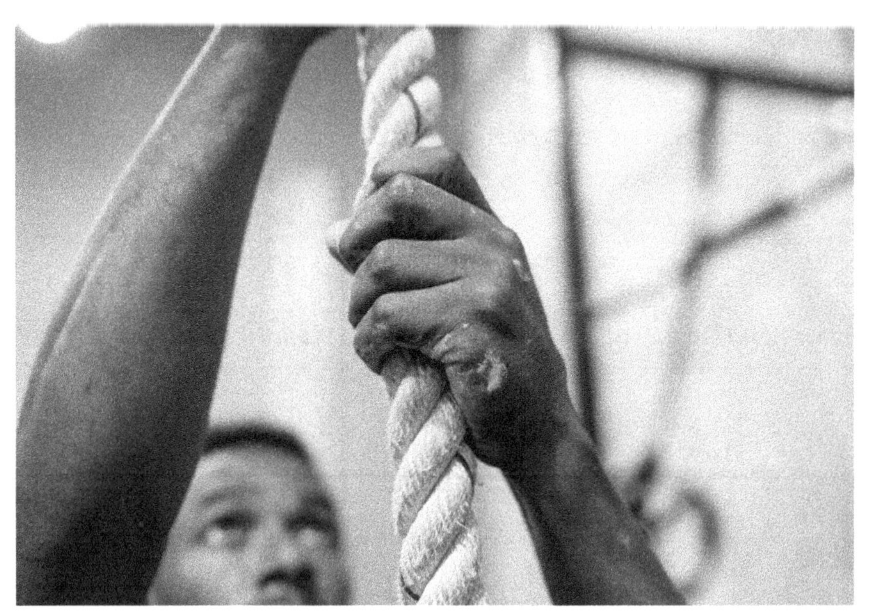

6

CrossFit At Any Age: What It Is, What It Ain't

"Over the long run, people don't stick to a workout regimen because of superhuman willpower—they stick with it because they realize how much better they feel after a workout. Sweat = Bliss. This is a universal neurobiological fact. Breaking a sweat is a hedonic pursuit."

—Dr. Christopher Bergland

Is CrossFit okay for 60-somethings? Absolutely! Can it hurt you? Heck yeah, if you're not ready to do the exercises or if you overexert during workouts. This will also happen in every sport and exercise regimen out there.

As the last chapter explained, the most important thing for us 60-somethings is to be well prepared before starting, because our body is not the same as it was at 20 when we were bulletproof and thought life would never end.

The Best Thing That Ever Happened To You

CrossFit, when applied correctly over time, can be the best thing to ever happen to you, especially as you hit 61. High-intensity interval and intermittent training is what our body was engineered for. Just so you know: interval training or exercising involves "resting" following burst activity. When you rest in interval work, you don't actually stop, you just slow to a walk or gentle movement.

In intermittent work, your rest period is an actual stop. After a sprint, you stop for a period of time, then resume your sprint. The two produce different results in your body: interval work burns more fat and improves endurance more. Intermittent work is less taxing on the body and produces smaller results but it's still very effective in your exercise routine.

Like our ape progenitors, humans excel at doing burst activities like sprinting, relaxing for a longer period of time, then doing another round of high-intensity work, like catching runaway bananas and mangos. They practiced intermittent routines.

Ever watch a day in the life of a cat? Sleeeeep. Rouse to stretch. Walk around the house, see what's up. Nibble on kibbles. Back to bed for some more sleeeeep. Cats love intermittent work, too.

We're kinda like cats, though we do need to take a break from 18 hours of chillaxin' to go to a regular job each day. The stop-and-go approach forces the body to react to a load placed on it, and the body must also react to the sudden, often unexpected acceleration required to complete the movement.

"CrossFit is *anabolic* and *kinetic*. With moderate-intensity exercise plus tabatas, it physically and chemically builds muscle and all the supporting organs, tissues, and cell cycles to create a bigger, better, faster you who will endure more!"

That type of shock to the body causes the release of hundreds of different hormones, cofactors, antioxidants, neurotransmitters, and other chemicals in and outside the central nervous system, all of which serve thousands of duties that improve your fitness.

Some prepare the body for stress. Others order muscles and tendons to spring into action, without overexerting them. Others direct the limbs to act in coordination with the trunk and core, ensuring smooth movements and actions.

Some send calming messages to the brain so we don't get too anxious or overexert ourselves. And, of course, many types of endorphins serve to make us feel high and ecstatic, and at the same time dull the pain so we can continue our work without interruption.

Endorphins and similar molecules produce those euphoric highs that serve to cheer us on and encourage us to *move*. And they deliver those benefits at just the right concentration, frequency and duration, without overdoing it or later producing deleterious effects like withdrawals.

CrossFit and its attendant exercises and routines all act as one to give our body the fullest workout possible in the shortest time, usually an hour at a time, once a day. When we crossfit, we are just following the laws of our genetic language, which codes for long, sustained work, punctuated with many short bursts of intense activity.

The Benefits Of CrossFit Extend Into The Next Day

It's perfectly fine to crossfit for an hour, then go about your daily routine for the rest of the day or evening. Longer than an hour may produce more delayed-onset soreness than you can handle. An hour allows the body to recover sufficiently for 48 hours. I've found that, say, two hours at a time makes me too sore and very tired. I go home for a three-hour siesta and miss half the day. Nope, my advice is that you do no more than an hour of CrossFit each session.

The healthful effects following your CrossFit workout extend well into days that overlap subsequent workouts, increasing the overall effect and its benefits.

Thus, the effects become cumulative and your body puts those effects to good use, to prepare your body for an uptick in your level of activity: it builds stronger muscles, tendons, ligaments; its metabolism increases; it moves harmful chemicals from the body through bowel and kidney elimination and also perspiration; it sequesters deleterious molecules in the liver and specific cellular organelles of other organs; plus many other still-unknown benefits.

The Neanderthals Developed Proto-CrossFit

Evolutionarily, it is a life of smooth movements and tiny mad minutes that combine to keep us alert and ready for the unexpected. Our ancestors didn't "work out" for many hours a day. They did mild to moderate workouts most of the day, with small increments of mad exercise (read: running from a lion).

Our foredads and foremoms discovered that prolonged workouts were bad for business and they led to an uncomfortable life or an early grave. Also, burning the midnight oil was not in our early evolutionary program. Our ancestors knew the importance of deep sleep.

Is "The Competition" Really Competition?

As with everything in life, there will come a new workout technique that somehow benefits us even more than CrossFit, but we've yet to see it. I don't discount the new machines and high-tech gadgets touted by fitness gurus, but I much prefer a simpler workout using what CrossFit offers.

Besides, to adequately wake up and exercise those stabilizer muscles, you must use free weights. High-tech doesn't cut it there. Recall what Occam told us hundreds of years ago: the simplest explanation (or action) is often the correct one.

Sure, I tried out several of the new million-dollar gyms in my area, and was blown away by all those unused fancy machines. In the end, some people felt like I do: *CrossFit* rocks!

The naysayers, though, heavily criticize CrossFit for causing many undue injuries because of "dangerous movements," "inappropriate levels of intensity," and for permitting unqualified people to coach CrossFit sessions.

What those same critics conveniently omit from their reports are the many other physical activities that cause even worse harm, and do so consistently. Ever heard of motocross? Cheerleading? Skiiing? Gymnastics?

Friends in the know tell me that girls' gymnastics is the most dangerous sport in the world today.

Mountaineering causes thousands of injuries and many deaths each year, far more than any negative statistic produced by CrossFit.

Fact is, the injury rate from doing CrossFit is about the same as for any other fitness model, even yoga. Yes, yoga.

Another fact: CrossFit is *anabolic*. It physically and chemically builds muscle and all the supporting tissues, cell cycles, etc. that create a bigger, better, faster you who can endure more than the average person!

There is no better method of working out for me, and I've seen 'em all. Yoga included. Truth? I now love yoga, as well.

How Much CrossFit Is Too Much CrossFit?

A question I hear a lot: Is an hour of CrossFit too much at a time? As I said above, an hour is just right for doing CrossFit given its intensity.

During that hour, people incorrectly assume that you have to go full afterburner for 60 minutes. Not true. For us 60-something crossfitters, we can scale each workout to our own body.

If we can't do 10 sets of deadlifts at 70% of our max, then we scale down to a doable level and perform there. If we can't run, then we get on a rower and pedal the same distance, if not farther.

In time, you'll decide if you are gonna *train* at a competitive level and maybe go to local, regional and national events, or *exercise* for fun and fitness, and be a spectator at CrossFit events.

Me? I'm having entirely too much fun just *exercising* and feeling great after each workout. That stored energy keeps building up the more I exercise, and lasts for days and propels me through my other work and play. Paradoxically, that same high energy ensures I sleep well at night and without interruption.

At my CrossFit box, I do sometimes compete against the other crossfitters on an occasional weekend, but those little competitions are few and far between. The camaraderie and competition are fun for me only in the short term.

I've found that, at 61, training takes too much out of me and I don't enjoy the workouts nearly as much. You may feel different about it, though, so try it out for yourself, see how it treats you.

During normal CrossFit classes, my coach has me doing double the distance on the rower that my peers run on the track outside. CrossFit is tailored to *my* level of fitness, and allows me to improve and build with each week of work.

Again, I'm not training to be the next Mat Fraser. Chris Winter is having loads of fun doing his own level of CrossFit, and he feels like a million bucks doing it.

Consider This: Private CrossFit Sessions

I also do at least one 30-minute private session of CrossFit each week with my favorite coach. After doing that for six months, I found that 30 minutes was perfect for doing supplementary exercises and working on my techniques for each CrossFit movement.

In those private sessions, he has me working my *stabilizer* muscles in my shouders, something I never even heard of before CrossFit. I now have shoulders that are bigger, stronger and more flexible than ever before.

My movements in everything I do are smoother, not kind of jerky like before. Bless those little-known stabilizer muscles in all the major muscle groups. I had no idea these guys existed until my coach had me doing special exercises to develop the stabilizers.

Example: I sit under a 45-lb. barbell and my coach hangs 10-lb. dumbbells off the ends of the barbell, each suspended from one of those colored rubber workout bands. I then do strict presses, pushing up those wobbly ends until I can push without wobble.

It takes a lot of practice to wake up and exercise the stabilizers in my shoulders, but when they are properly awakened and exercised, I'm able to do much better strict presses (and other barbell and dumbbell exercises) without the rubber bands.

The effect is really disconcerting at first, when I'm using the dumbbells suspended from the bands. But when I get the hang of it, I discover a whole new tool for exercising and lifting. These unique stabilizer exercises enable me (and you!) to lift more and have much better control during regular weightlifting. Amazing!

Something else I truly love and am completely addicted to: the loud, intense 60-minute CrossFit sessions with a group of like-minded crossfitters. The energy is infectious and lasts days that easily carry into the next week. Physicists tell us that perpetual motion is impossible. All the benefits of CrossFit prove otherwise.

They complement each other well, the private training and the regular CrossFit classes. Plus, my coach is right there to guide me, coach me, and correct me when I'm out of focus. That kind of immediate feedback makes a better, safer and happier crossfitter.

What Really Is "Fit"?

As I explained in Chapter 4, the term "fit" is far from having a "one size fits all" definition. It's really an artificial term invented by some clever marketing people in some high-rise to sell a lotta products like food, athletic apparel, basketball shoes, etc. And it has also programmed millions of people into thinking their way.

Fit has a thousand different meanings and only applies to each individual person. A fun fact: our own US government's guidelines cannot adequately define "fit" on any level, either, because they include in their definition only the categories and bullet points they see as important.

I know hundreds of fit people who do not do CrossFit or any organized form of exercise, yet they're the ones who live well past 100 years. Putting it simply, fit is whatever you make it, especially if you feel good every day, are healthy, and have a good sense of well-being. That said, you can still enjoy crossfitting yourself, too!

"No Pain, No Gain" Is Beyond Stupid

It hurts! And it causes serious injuries. Always has.

CrossFitters who used to do pure weightlifting in traditional gyms said they were injured more there than doing CrossFit. The old saying is from the 1970s when guys like Arnold YouKnowWho promoted the abuse of anabolic steroids, human growth hormone, consuming pounds of beef and eggs a day, and preached "no pain-no gain" like unlettered Southern Baptists.

No wonder Olympic weightlifting got a bad rap, and it wasn't even Arnold and Gang's method of training. Those guys used to poo-poo Olympic weightlifting.

CrossFit promotes smart exercise and does not condone the use of any performance-enhancing drugs or fad diets. You don't need illicit drugs to crossfit yourself into shape. CrossFit itself is a drug that acts on many levels, and you have to experience it first hand to appreciate this fact.

What I've Discovered After A Year Of CrossFit

I have no pulled muscles, no tired and achy muscles; no torn ligaments; no torn or strained tendons; no lousy moods upon waking up from a deep sleep; no unpleasant thoughts, in general; no constipation; and no feeling of discomfort.

Instead, CrossFit leaves me with well-worked muscles that are limber and warm; stronger ligaments and tendons; much greater flexibility and range of motion; uplifted moods; steady sleep patterns; great thoughts and feelings of well-being; regular bowel movements; more stable blood glucose levels and other biomarkers of great physical health; no diseases or general aches and pains from being sedentary.

I'm still working on my diet, but I find myself preparing more salads and eating lots of fruits, and drinking a gallon or more of distilled water each day. I consciously avoid junk food and drinks, and no longer have a mild craving for either.

It's as if some inner voice is calling for this better diet. I know my body has specific enteroreceptors that allow me to somehow sense some of the many physiological processes going on inside my body. I can actually sense an "entity" that is asking me for fruits and veggies. Another voice used to ask me for sugary foods. While it is not totally silent, that demon voice is very small and insignificant.

That is the biggest breakthrough I've had since starting CrossFit: seeing and feeling a change in my diet. Like I said earlier, I still struggle with it, and it's a work in progress.

Are my gut microbes directing me to eat better foods? Slowly, yes. But they still have to do battle with my bad microbes, which rear their ugly heads once in a while and call for a Dr Pepper or some ice cream.

Confession: I'm also feeling great now because of a choice I made before I started. And it was simple: exercise, don't train. I was determined to find a happy medium between the two, knowing the benefits of both.

I knew that moderate exercise was better than little to no exercise. Training was too intense for me, too, but I still could incorporate some of the Tabatas from training in my own routines.

By finding a comfortable space between exercising and training, I am a new man.

To top it off, I have new friends and colleagues who enjoy my company. I socialize more, in general, outside CrossFit, because my mood is so strongly positive.

No more staying inside all day to write a book or do some other project. I no longer have to drag myself outta bed and the house to do cool things and meet fun and energetic people.

CrossFit is my new superpower.

Watch out! It may become *yours*, too!

After a year of CrossFit and 60+ years experiencing life, I developed a hypothesis about the various stages of health and fitness. It's much more involved than this, of course, but this simplified continuum clearly spells out your five main options:

THE ENDLESS CONTINUUM OF FITNESS

Sedentary Lifestyle = Poor Fitness, Early Death

Mild Exercise = Feel Better

Moderate Exercise = Good Fitness and Health

Moderate Exercise + Tabatas =
Excellent Life-Long Health, Fitness and Well-Being

Daily High-Intensity Interval Training =
Short-Term Good Health + Long-Term Damage

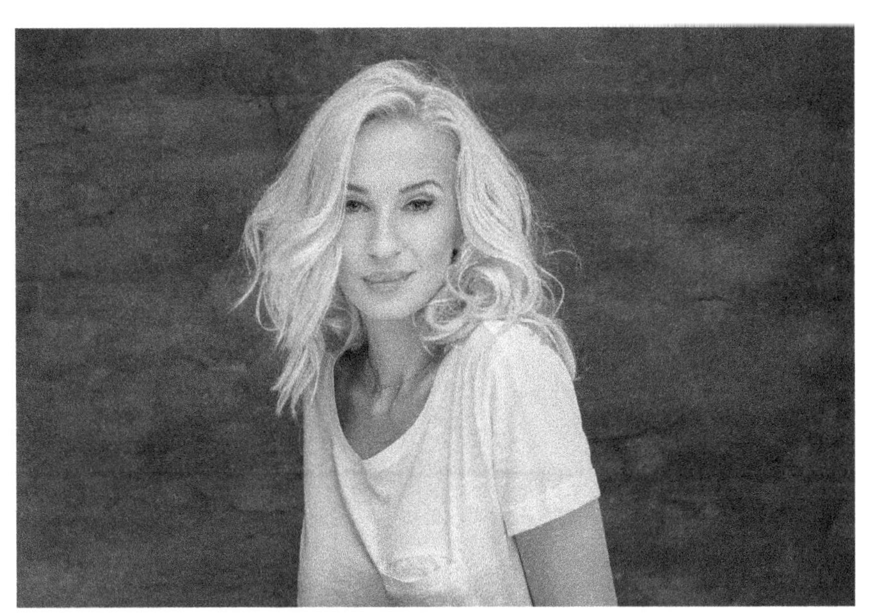

7

61 Is The New 41

"Before I discovered CrossFit, I was an avid potato-coucher who would watch every sports event on tv. The only reasons I got up: pee, grab the next beer, a coupla Snickers, and bag of Doritos."

—[Honestly, I forgot]

Seems everywhere we look these days, we see sexy, physically fit, coiffed-out, silver-haired souls who look absolutely fabulous in their glowing skin. These are the middle-agers struttin' into CrossFit boxes all over America, not to mention high-rise offices, restaurants and bars, black-tie events, Publix, Home Depot, Trader Joe's, World Market, etc.

You've probably seen a few, maybe even been impressed by their high level of fitness, poise, strength and humility. Maybe you've even wondered how they got that way, and felt a little envious.

I Love Meeting New People. You Should, Too!

Me? Whenever I spot one of these beautiful souls, I walk up to them and chat 'em up, compliment them, ask them what they eat for breakfast, what they do for work, how they're enjoying life. The response I've always gotten first is a huuuge smile, followed by a gracious thank you! I've been fortunate in life: not one single person I've chatted up rebuffed me. Ever.

I've asked many of these people how they felt before CrossFit:

shitty! And then after a year of CrossFit: Wao! Clearly, something positive is going on in the lives of those who choose CrossFit as a new lifestyle. It's not a cult, mind you. It is a new way of living and enjoying life.

Look Great Naked!

Many 60+ women are turning the heads of 20- and 30-something men—some even keeping a few boy-toys, I hear—and they're doing it in skin-tight tops and dresses that would've given the Greatest Generation a five-alarm stroke.

The athletes defining this new elite class look every bit 41 years old as, well, 41-year-old girls. Plus, they have the wisdom and grace their younger peers have yet to achieve, and those added traits elevate our 60-something beauties to a whole new level others cannot touch. Yet.

I did an informal examination on Match.com, and looked strictly at those women over 60. Surprisingly, more than half were looking for men in their 30s and 40s!

Some even in their 20s, and they weren't shy about stating their interest, often in bold capital letters that served to warn off anyone who didn't fit their strict preferences.

Gawd, I swear those women had bigger cojones than any guy I knew. Actually, that's a silly statement and it brings to mind a joke I heard from actress Betty White:

"We shouldn't say 'grow a pair of balls!' Those things are so fragile and delicate. We should be saying, '*Grow a vagina!*', 'cos those things take a pounding!"

I contacted several of them and couldn't even reach them because they'd set the age range much lower than my 60 years. Wao, good for them.

As an aside, when I lived in the Bahamas years ago, there was a secret society of wealthy women who had these weekend parties that featured young men around 20-something.

I talked with one of those women and she told me, "You only live once, Chris, so go for exactly what you want and never ever settle for less."

Oh, I'm not sure whether those older women were actively doing CrossFit, but something tells me they probably couldn't fit it onto their dance cards.

Not sure about May-December romances among highly fit 60+ men and younger women but—not to sound at all suggestive here—I do pray they exist.

61 is, indeed, the new 41, and CrossFit gets a lot of the credit.

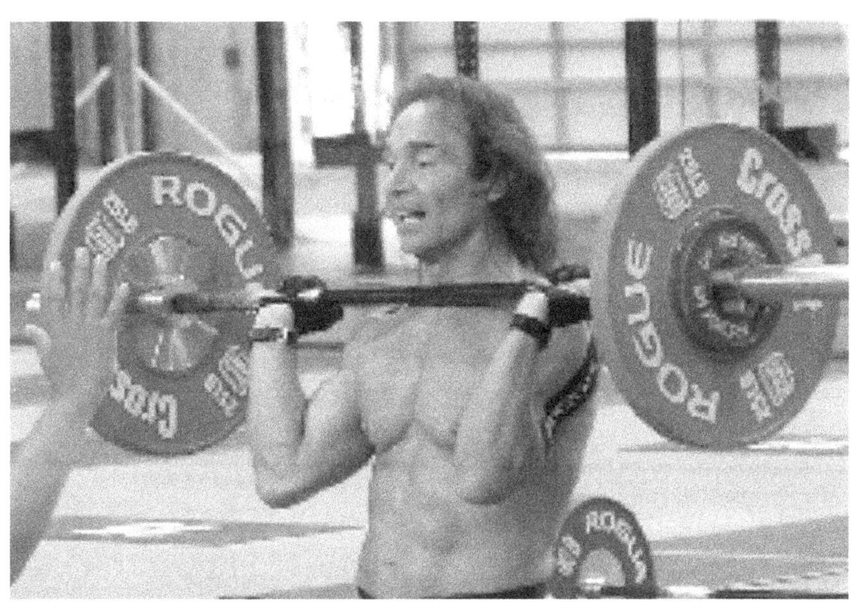

An Intimate Chat with Elite CrossFitter Dr. Dave Hippensteel

"I really want my life to be an example of encouragement and inspiration to those struggling with anxiety and depression, and inspire them to move in a direction of fitness. "

—Dr. Dave Hippensteel

Thank goodness for wonderful and approachable elite crossfitters like Dave Hippensteel and Armando Besne, two of my CrossFit heroes who set a great example for the rest of us, even though we may not wanna train like they do.

Again, there's a huge difference between exercising and training. These two men train hard. I include their stories here because they may inspire some to pursue training for competitions.

For those like me, they are for entertainment purposes.

This and the next chapter feature the wisdom and experience of these wonderful human beings who, in their sixties, have killed it at several different CrossFit Games, coming in first and second place, respectively.

Dave Hippensteel Shares His Story

I'm thinking, probably the most ironic thing about my story personally is that I hated sports growing up. My parents forced me to play sports and I really rebelled against it for a while.

But as times changed, so did I and it was actually sports that saved me from a very destructive direction I'd chosen for myself early on in my wild and crazy high school years.

I remember very vividly one day looking in the mirror after a series of traumatic experiences and saying to myself, "Why am I trying to destroy the body God gifted me?"

And from that point on, I started on a journey of profound change in my life and committed to move in the direction of excellence, not only when it comes to health, but also intellectually and spiritually.

At 155 pounds and after a very successful high school football career, I wanted to play in college but was injured very soon during the first several weeks of football camp.

So with a severely sprained neck and no football I decided to study the books for the first time in my life, and amazingly found success there, as well.

It was fun having something to excel in and meet the demands of a rigorous academic schedule. Thinking for at least a short period of time my sports career was over, I found myself the next year on the track team at Cal State Fresno doing the decathlon with my older brother, who was always dreaming of going to the Olympics one day.

> "I was determined to practice squatting for hours every night for probably three years, and every year my squat mobility got better."

Training for the decathlon every day I got in such awesome shape that I think this was the first time I reinforced an inner desire and commitment to be in the best shape of my life as a lifelong quest.

You see, one of the healthiest decisions I think we can make is becoming passionate about being in the best shape of our lives, because it just feels right and the benefits in life are almost innumerable!

Think about this: no one wakes up in the morning and says I wish I wasn't in great shape. We're always wishing the opposite, right? And if you develop the right habits of fitness, it will stay with you and serve you well for a lifetime.

After college was dental school, where it was really tough to balance academics and exercise, I managed to stay in shape at least on occasion so I never lost my fitness altogether.

After dental school I asked myself, "What can I do next to challenge myself physically?" and the only thing I knew of was the triathlon because I knew I just didn't wanna run as much as I loved it, I wanted to learn and be challenged by a multi-disciplined sport.

For the next 20 years, off and on, I raced triathlons, mostly Olympic distance and some sprint-distance tri's. It was also during this time that we raised four awesome kids who are all grown now but all have caught the vision of fitness for life!

When I turned 40, I decided there was another sport that I always really wanted to do: race motocross. I started out racing Enduros and hare scrambles and eventually got on the motocross track with huge jumps and loved every second of it. I raced for about five years and had a track in my backyard with several 60-foot jumps and one 90-foot jump I used to hit routinely.

We ended up moving to Tennessee to work an old musical passion of mine: guitar and song writing. I got away from dirt biking and I started playing lots of soccer and coaching the kids' soccer teams. It was a fun sport to enjoy with the kids those years and kept us all in great shape until I discovered CrossFit about 10 years later.

Motocross and triathlons and soccer kept me quite fit over those decades, but when I discovered CrossFit I experienced a whole other level of fitness. It seemed to rival the fitness I had achieved doing decathlon those years back in college and it felt like all the energy, stamina, strength and endurance I had as a college-age decathlete I had resurrected somehow in the sport of CrossFit.

There was no turning back and I committed to one absolutely dialed-in focus: winning gold medals in CrossFit.

I won the first open I ever actually trained for, in 2013. I went to the games that year and ended up in fifth place, which most people thought was an amazing accomplishment, because I had only been doing CrossFit for about a year.

I still left with a bit of a disappointment for not winning, though. It should have been the thrill of a lifetime to be in the top five in the world, but for me there was no rest and no break. It was back to training the next week after games with a constant pursuit of perfection in this new sport I had come to embrace as my new calling in life.

My issues or challenges were never related to strength or agility. That for me has always been a given but there were definitely mobility issues that I had to overcome to be the best in the world. So I worked at it relentlessly, day in and day out. I soon realized it was full squats and hip mobility that I needed to perfect.

I was determined to practice squatting for hours every night for probably three years and every year my squat mobility got better. And along with that, my competitiveness grew and finally after only three years competing in the sport I achieved my first gold medal in 2016, winning the first event and maintaining the lead the entire three days with three total wins and a victory over second place by more than 50 points.

It was a real sense of achievement and exactly what I had worked so hard for all those years. But as satisfying as it was, I set my sights on the next year and worked even harder, breaking down each individual skill and discipline so no weaknesses would be exposed. Once again I came away with the victory with even a much more competitive field than the prior year.

Now, you would think that would be enough: two gold medals. I have to admit, it's one of the greatest experiences of my life. However soon after that gold medal I started thinking about the next year and how nice it would be to taste victory one more time and so the quest began, and again in 2018 I came away with a solid win and a third gold medal.

The year 2019 will definitely be a year to remember for many reasons: I had applied and been accepted to the show Ninja Warrior, so while I was training and qualifying for my seventh CrossFit Games and 4th year in the age group, I was also preparing for a Ninja Warrior competition.

Somehow it ended up being a bit too much for my body to handle and that year became riddled with injuries: first, a severe calf strain during the qualifier, then a groin pull, and then two weeks before the

2019 games I herniated two discs in my lower back (L4-L5 area), but stubbornly refused to stop even though hindsight says I should have. Miraculously that year I still managed to come away with a fifth place finish my fourth year into the age group.

About a month after the games, I was facing the possibility of surgery on my lower back. I figured my career in Crossfit was finished. And then the unexpected happened: I started feeling better without surgery and so I got back in the gym and did what I could do to maintain fitness while still allowing my back to heal.

"I like to say that CrossFit has given me a second wind in life."

And even though the Crossfit Open for the first time ever was in the fall instead of spring, I was healed enough and felt well enough to be able to compete in the Crossfit Open and clawed my way back from 170th in the first event all the way up to 8th overall after five events. By the time the online qualifier came around, I was fully healed and back in great shape and once again managed to qualify for what would become my eighth year in competition.

When it came time for the online qualifier, I had no idea that my fifth year in the age group, coming back from a back injury just six months before, would pay off so well. I shocked myself and I think much of the CrossFit world by finishing in the top three and solidly qualifying for my eight year at the Crossfit Games.

But the very next week, right after the online qualifier, covid hit and within two months the Masters competition was canceled. So I thought once again my career must be over, or maybe this was a sign that I need to take off, maybe find another sport, or just take a break completely.

Little did I know that is not how the story ends.

The Masters fitness collective said it wasn't fair that the masters athletes were not competing, so they decided to bring the masters CrossFit games championship back and it got scheduled as a live event for August 2020.

I was thrilled but a bit apprehensive as to whether or not this would actually come to fruition, but once again I continued to dream and visualize another gold medal and a huge comeback, and redemption from the previous year's injury.

When the workouts came out, it looked to me like quite a few of them were not that well balanced for true CrossFit Games testing. There was a part of me that wanted to say, "Now it's over, no reason to continue, you've got three gold medals, you don't need to prove anything, you can stop now."

But that's never how I've lived my life, and so once again I found myself on the starting line of that first event and by the end of the first day I was on my way probably to the greatest accomplishment of my CrossFit career, because when you're five years into the age group you're not supposed to win, let alone win by over 100 points.

After four days and nine events total, which made it the most grueling of all of the eight years, I achieved yet another gold medal and attained a near-perfect record in the 60+ age division for all five years.

What does the next year hold? We will see. . . .

Did your parents or mentors give you advice about how to live life at age 60+?

I would say yes, in that my dad especially stayed active all the way into his 90s. So in that sense, he was a real example of how beneficial it is to keep yourself *moving* into your later years. I think that's why he lived so long and healthy all of his life.

My parents always encouraged me to do sports growing up so although I wasn't really happy about it in the beginning, I came to really appreciate the level of fitness I achieved by being in sports such as football and track, all of my growing up years.

How did you keep in great shape after age 60?

Ever since high school and especially in college where I did decathlon and learned what it was like to be in the absolute best shape of my life, I kind of kept that going into my sixties.

After college and dental school, doing triathlons and then

eventually discovered CrossFit, which has taken me through the last ten years and has really upped the level of my fitness overall. I think that contributes to internal health, as well. This commitment to fitness over my lifetime has set me up really well for maintaining that fitness into my later years.

How did you discover CrossFit? Why did you fall in love with it?

So, my daughter first introduced me to CrossFit around 2011-2012. She knew I would love it because we were always a fit family and always doing pull ups and stuff like that.

She grew up as a gymnast and then became a college diver so through her encouragement I checked out a local gym and also checked out the gym where she was training.

I immediately fell in love with CrossFit because of the versatility it offered in testing you in so many dimensions of physical fitness. I've always been kind of strong for my size and had a knack for gymnastics but never got to really test those sports. So the combination of Olympic lifting and gymnastics was like a match made in heaven for me.

I always wanted to do gymnastics as a kid but missed out on it because we didn't have a local team and my dad wanted me to play football, so the closest I got was doing pole vault in the decathlon in college.

I think doing decathlon in college was where I first realized there's a level of fitness you achieve when you work on all three of your energy systems, which is what we do in CrossFit.

What has CrossFit done for you?

I like to say that CrossFit has given me a second wind in life because there're not a whole lot of choices to compete when you turn 50 or 60, except for maybe triathlons or just running.

But that's really not gonna get you the fitness that's ideal for your joints and overall health and longevity.

So for me it opened up the door to understand the relationship between fitness health and longevity.

Through CrossFit I discovered the relationship between being really fit and having healthy blood biomarkers, those measurable things [blood pressure, glucose, etc.] in your body that determine your level of health [at that moment] and ultimate longevity.

What's your diet?

I decided to try Paleo the first year I started doing CrossFit, just because the most fit guys in the gym were doing that. So I thought I'd give it a try. I immediately fell in love with how it made me feel.

Even though I had been eating a healthy diet with lots of grains, vegetables and some meat, and racing triathlons, what I experienced with Paleo and CrossFit took me to a whole new level of fitness!

I really like simplicity. With my career, there're so many decisions to make. Honestly, I don't mind not having choices for breakfast, lunch or dinner so I don't mind eating the same thing every single day.

My diet is pretty simple: I have meat, avocado and spinach for lunch and breakfast and then I mix it up at dinner with sometimes more vegetables like asparagus, broccoli maybe carrots, celery or kale or even cabbage.

For snacks, I always go to almonds and cashews and sometimes walnuts and sunflower seeds. It's a super healthy snack with no downside.

Do you also do yoga?

Stretching is a huge factor and yoga has been helpful but my brother has his own version of stretching program that he developed himself and it is the absolute most comprehensive stretching/ mobility routine on the planet.

In fact he actually got mentioned in Dave Goggins book, *Can't Hurt Me: Master Your Mind and Defy the Odds*, because he'd helped Dave get his life back through his stretching program.

It's hard to take the time to do the stretching routine with my very busy schedule with CrossFit and dentistry, but when I do I see the benefits, especially when it helped me recover from a severe double-herniated disc back injury in 2019.

Do you get regular deep-tissue or sports massages?

My success over the last eight or nine years is due in a large part to my massage therapists I see on a regular basis, and also Arosti which is the group of chiropractors who do deep tissue at the CrossFit Games. For the last eight years, I've learned more and more from them.

They've helped me through many an event at the Games, including making sure that I could follow through in 2016 when I had a severe abdominal strain. I needed to finish strong to keep the lead and win my first gold medal. I really believe I could not have finished strong without their help.

Do you use nutritional supplements?

I'm really fortunate to be sponsored by the company Inside Tracker, a blood analysis company mainly for athletes. They help get you dialed in for your nutritional needs by identifying any deficiencies in your biomarkers.

Based on a lot of the recommendations, I take supplements including vitamin C, vitamin D. I do take creatine, as well, another one of their recommendations.

They also help me connect with a supplement company. I love being supported by them: Klean Athlete. They've been supplying me with my supplements for several years now and are always making sure I'm getting the vitamins and minerals I need to sustain optimal fitness.

Also another awesome company who gives me most of my protein is Ascent. Protein has been a huge factor. I don't think I could eat all the protein I need without their supply of extra protein I need to build and maintain muscle.

Also another company I've been working with over the the last year is Vital Proteins. They, too, are an awesome company and their CEO Kurt has discovered how essential collagen is for our bodies as we age.

How do you stay healthy mentally?

I believe that physical and mental health exist on a continuum, meaning everyone has a predisposition to move the needle in either direction. You can be depressed and anxious, or be optimistic and mentally healthy and sharp, upbeat and happy, content, grateful, all those good things that exist on the right side of the scale.

I think every day we all battle with which direction we are going to move on that continuum. CrossFit has definitely helped me keep the balance in mental physical and emotional health and move the needle continually in the direction of greater joy, contentment and fulfillment in my life, and away from destruction.

I really want my life to be an example of encouragement and inspiration to those who are struggling with anxiety and depression, and help inspire them to move in a direction of fitness, because it has a huge impact on their emotional, mental and spiritual health.

I believe, and this is a huge topic for another day, but I really think that our spiritual dimension plays a big role also in our emotional and mental health and well-being.

We are eternal beings and it's important to have eternity settled in our minds and hearts to live healthy and balanced life here and now.

I had my spiritual awakening in my early 20s, and I really feel like it has been a huge part in carrying me through all of the challenges this life throws at us.

What do you wish to say to those approaching 60?

OMG! What can I say, but train hard, train to live. We were born for this physiologically! We are designed to benefit from healthy exercise and healthy eating and there're severe consequences for ignoring that.

It's why we are having the epidemic of chronic disease in our country and most of the world right now and have for decades. If I ever get the time or opportunity, I would love to be on a mission to tell my story, either through a book or speaking tour, or even through a health retreat or a CrossFit-type training camp.

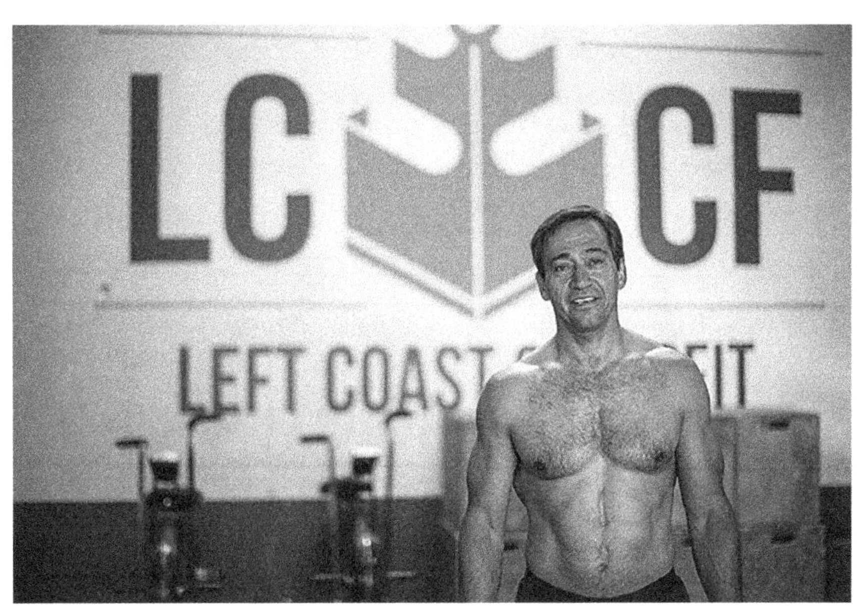

9

An Intimate Chat with Elite CrossFitter Armando Besne

"I didn't start CrossFit to be a competitor.
I just wanted to stay healthy."
—Armando Besne

My parents and I immigrated from Mexico City in 1966 when I was nine years old. We first settled in the suburbs of Los Angeles and I didn't speak any English. The school system did not offer an ESL program back then, so it was total immersion in the language and culture.

Looking back now, I feel grateful since that's the best way to learn a language. However, I had to overcome a lot of obstacles at school, in and out of the classroom. My schoolmates had a quite a few bruises and so did I.

Back then, the school held an annual National Presidential Fitness Test that involved the broad jump, sit-ups, and pull-ups from what I vaguely remember. That's when I realized I had some athletic ability.

I was watching the 1968 Olympics held in Mexico City on a black and white TV, and was amazed by this American high jumper who had a very different technique. Instead of the forward "western roll," he jumped over the bar backwards.

I couldn't wait to try this myself.

Inspired and determined, the kids in my neighborhood hung a

rope between two trees and put a mattress underneath so that we could all practice. This went on for months. Pretty soon I was doing the famous Fosbury Flop.

In high school, I ran varsity cross-country, played soccer, and was also on the swim team. I excelled very quickly in swimming and was always one to focus on technique.

Don't be afraid to try new things!

Don't let self-doubt be an obstacle, because you might surprise yourself!

After my college years, I enlisted in the Marine Corps and maintained my physical health well beyond that by running, lifting weights and swimming. I never stopped working out because I truly enjoy being healthy.

Health is wealth, as we all know.

My first CrossFit workout was initiated by my wife. She was intrigued by the sign outside of a box: "Look better naked."

For the record, she already looked great naked!

She signed up for the "on-ramp" classes, and I went with her out of curiosity. The coach challenged me to join in, but I was totally unprepared, still in jeans.

The workout of the day, or WOD, consisted of air squats, pull-ups, and push-ups. The Coach asked if I was in shape, and I said yes. After all, I kept myself fit all these years, or so I thought.

Also joining us in the WOD was a very slender woman with very skinny arms. The Coach pointed to her and said: "Try to keep up with her."

Suffice it to say, the skinny-armed woman and the WOD kicked my butt!

I immediately signed up and did my first CrossFit Games Open a year later.

Why did I fall in love with CrossFit?

I like the variety and challenge of each WOD. I like the fact that it combines all the different disciplines: gymnastics, lifting, running, etc. I enjoy learning new skills.

So, what has CrossFit done for me?

It makes me feel young. I feel mentally and physically strong. It's my fountain of youth and gives me that playful feeling I had as a youngin' on the playground. It's vital to my sense of well-being.

I don't follow a special diet but I believe in clean healthy foods and limited simple sugars. Some carbs are good. I will eat pizza, but it won't be covered in cheese. Veggie pizza is my go-to.

Candy bars, cakes, donuts, etc. are non-existent in my diet. So, it's not a special diet per se, just low in sugars. Throw that Snickers bar in the trash and eat an apple with peanut butter instead.

As far as preparation for a workout, it tends to be the same every time: strong bourbon, a cigarette, and a quicky do the trick every time. Just kidding. :)

A half-hour of light stretching, catching up on gym gossip, rolling on the ol' foam roller is necessary to loosen the rust.

Additional rolling and stretching post-WOD for a cool-down.

When I competed, I got regular massages, but now my wife does it. Yes, she still looks good naked!

As far as supplements go, whey protein, branched-chain amino acids (BCAA), and electrolytes are all I take in. I am not on any prescription medications, nor do I plan to get on them. I definitely don't believe in performance-enhancing supplements.

My message to people in their 60s: exercise is vital to living life fully, and CrossFit is the perfect venue to do so. It allows you to start at any level of fitness.

I didn't start CrossFit to be a competitor. I just wanted to stay healthy. It elevated my level of fitness to such a degree that I thought *Why not go for it?* I eventually found myself competing at the Games in 2017 and again in 2018, finishing 6th and 2nd respectively.

It doesn't matter how many articles one reads, the motivation has to come from within. Self-motivation is critical to changing your life. Do you feel worthy to make a difference for yourself, to change your life for the better?

Too many older people get depressed and give up. CrossFit makes me feel like the best person I can be, so get off the couch and join me and the awesome community of CrossFit!

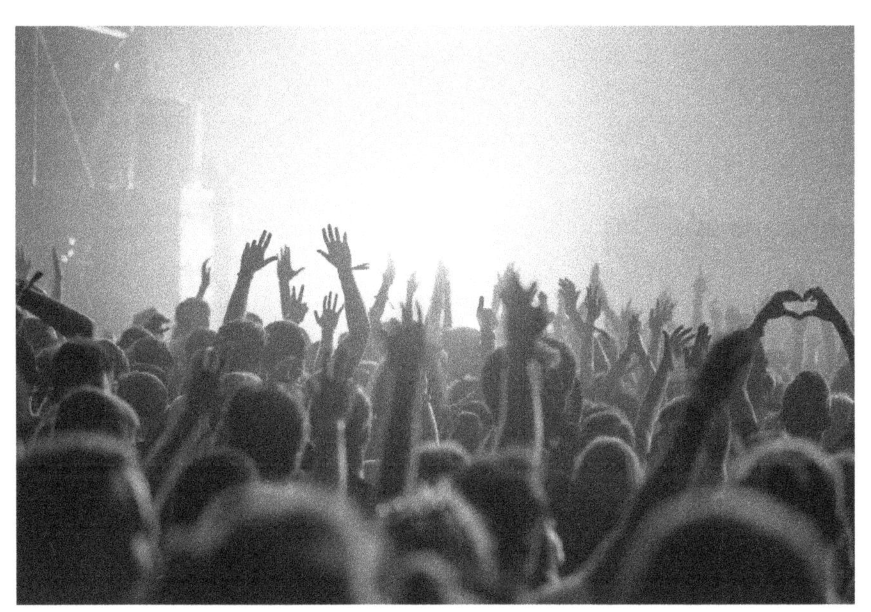

10

An Intimate Chat with 60+ CrossFitters Rachel, Lynda and Bobby. Oh, and Chris!

"CrossFit is a long-term program, but it's treated like a fast-food craze. That's why so many people try it and quit, or they never go at all."

—Rachel G

I spoke with many 60+ CrossFit athletes, four of whom agreed to share their experiences with me. I also threw in my own adventures in crossfitting at age 61. These athletes are not training for the CrossFit Games or any other competition. They exercise to feel great, to improve their overall health, and they pace themselves so they can exercise for life.

Powerful Rachel G Kills It!

Rachel G is a 62-year-old woman, an attorney in Florida, never married (except to her cool job), travels extensively, and who devotes considerable time to exercising and studying up on her legal cases.

Rachel G tells us:

I've always been active, even as a baby. My mom had to chase me around just to get a diaper on me. I still have an issue with clothes! In high school, I ran cross country for four years and had a blast, but it took a toll on my knees so I opted out of running in college. Instead, I tried yoga and jogging lightly on a treadmill. I still use a treadmill but it's self-powered: Assault AirRunner. Kick ass!

At first, yoga looked so boring! I watched a group of women in my city over a week, because that is how I learn, by observing others first. Then I start off slowly and get a feel for it. There was no way I could run again, except on a treadmill, so I knew that yoga had to work for me, so I kept at it and found it to be very relaxing when I held poses for a long time.

I didn't know that yoga required such muscle strength! I was using muscles that I didn't know I had, even though I had been a runner for years. They told me that running requires many different muscle groups over uneven terrain, and that was good for me. But at the same time, it's not exercising the core muscles enough to build them up even more.

That's what's so bad about just doing running for exercise: it does not work the little, seemingly insignificant stabilizer muscles or core muscles. It is a repetitive movement that focuses on the legs. Some will disagree with me, but I proved it with myself for many years.

"Some gyms have specialized senior programs that start you out very slowly, usually using a pvc pipe in place of a barbell. They also use colored rubber bands for strength and conditioning of individual muscles and large muscle groups."

At the yoga studio where I train, an orthopedic surgeon suggested I add some weight training to my routine, to build up all my muscles. At the time, and this was in the mid-1980s, CrossFit had not been born but there were small gyms that emphasized "total-body workouts" that included doing interval training, mostly sprints.

That did it for me, doing many different exercises in an hour. Believe it or not, I kept doing that well into 2002 when all my friends suddenly discovered CrossFit. It was as if a bomb dropped right on our gym. And soon the place converted from its old configuration to a CrossFit box. There were only half a dozen CrossFit gyms in the US at that time, so it was a big thing for us to be one of the first to launch.

Now, in 2021, there are something like 15,000 CrossFit boxes! That's phenomenal for an exercise program many criticize as being too hard on the body.

My orthopedic surgeon says, "People sometimes have an unrealistic expectation when beginning an exercise regimen. They jump into it too quickly and rigorously, and they end up overtaxing their muscles and joints and they quit. Many feel that CrossFit encourages this type of behavior, where people try it too enthusiastically, get injured, then quit and never return.

I think CrossFit boxes should learn better techniques of bringing novices along slowly, like over a year, so they can ease into all the exercises. Most I've seen or heard about just throw new students into it and don't give them proper instruction.

Olympic weightlifting is a killer on people's shoulders, so they must train very slowly using only a PVC pipe or light barbell to start. And I mean they should do this for the first year alone, and then gradually add weight. CrossFit is a long-term program, but it is treated like a fast-food craze. That's why so many people try it and quit, or they never go at all.

My ortho surgeon also sends me these long emails with her wise thoughts and ideas for proper training. So far, she has guided me safely through this whole process of staying in great shape at my age.

I've noticed something very interesting at age 60: my peers' bodies are starting to break down because they only walk or do light exercises, including yoga. But those light workouts are not enough to sustain good muscle mass, strong joints, stable core, good stabilizer muscles, and an overall healthy body.

Only moderate to high-intensity interval training does this, and I've found that it is the best way to stay fit in my 60s and I hope well into my 70s and 80s.

I'm always asked, "But what about nutrition?"

I've always eaten healthful foods, but also indulged in meat and fish. I do not eat red meat every day, and only eat it maybe once a month. As I have aged, I've felt how red meat stays inside my intestines much longer than chicken, turkey or fish.

Fish basically just dissolves like toilet paper as it passes through your intestines. I stopped eating fish last year, though, because it's not sustainable and it's also filled with nanoplastics, mercury, dioxins, and many other terrible chemicals from industrial, commercial and residential run-off into the oceans.

Red meat is like hard and tight beef jerky, and it doesn't want to break apart enough for you to digest it properly, even though I chew my food well. For some reason, the human body isn't built to digest red meat very well, and I can feel this every time I eat a hamburger. It takes a whole work week to get it out of my system.

So I now eat mostly what I call "rich and dense salads." They have every kind of leafy lettuce, with an abundance of spinach, plus twenty different kinds of raw veggies like carrots, mushrooms, cucumbers, beets and more. I mix it all up in a huge bowl, add spices and dressing to taste, and munch on it for a few days.

> "I feel the most important thing is to *show up*."

I find it keeps well in the fridge for even a week, and it even tastes better as the week goes on because the spices and dressing and all ingredients mix and diffuse into each other so well.

I also eat heavy soups with 15 different beans and lentils, plus potatoes and carrots. I do the soups in a big crockpot that makes enough for a month. Gazpacho and goulash are my winter go-to meals.

Drinks? I avoid alcohol, period. It gives me headaches. There are no drugs in my life, only a few supplements that I know actually work because I've tested them over decades. Things like Vitamin C, sodium bicarbonate, etc. I do drink about a gallon of water every day, too.

Some people tell me that's impossible for them to do, but I tell them how I do it: I keep two gallons of water at my office at any one time, and many gallons at home, all chilled. I make ice tea by adding a big tea bag to a gallon container, let it sit overnight, then break it into two gallons of lighter tea. It is a good flavored water, essentially, and adds spice to my drinking life.

My advice to people interested in feeling and looking better? It's never too late to start, except maybe if you're on your deathbed. I suggest finding the nearest CrossFit gym (they like to call it "box" but I still call it a gym sometimes) and making an appointment to talk with one of their senior coaches who knows about seniors like us.

Some gyms have specialized senior programs that start you out very slowly, usually using a pvc pipe in place of a barbell. They also use colored rubber bands for strength and conditioning of individual muscles and large muscle groups. While most gyms will charge their members about $150/month for unlimited CrossFit training, ask them for discounts for seniors, veterans, first responders, teachers, government workers, etc.

If you don't ask, you won't get anything!

My requirement for attending a CrossFit gym is that I feel good about being there when I exercise and feel good about going there when I'm away from the gym. I must feel excited about it or I will not want to pay the monthly membership fee, nor will I want to attend classes there.

The chemistry between me and my coaches is paramount, too. I've found that most CrossFit coaches are great at what they do and they love coaching, so they are enthusiastic and energetic and make you feel a part of their family.

I feel the most important thing is to *show up*.

And please have reasonable expectations. I promise you this: if you stick with it for 6-9 months, you will see noticeable improvement in your looks, how you feel, and your blood chemistry. Remember to see your doctor before starting CrossFit, and get a baseline blood chemistry and urinalysis done.

If you are diabetic or have some other disease or health issue, tell your doctor you want to do CrossFit for seniors, and ask their advice. A good doctor will know about CrossFit and hopefully encourage you to begin your program. I hope to see more and more seniors doing CrossFit. Happy journeys!

From The Vivacious Lynda C To Your Ears

Lynda C is a 60-year-old mother of three grown children. She was not an athlete in high school, and she did not attend college, instead choosing to be a full-time mother. When her husband passed away suddenly four years ago from a heart attack, she jumped into action and asked all her friends and neighbors what she should do to get into shape.

Lynda C tells us:

When Ben died, I was devastated and could not even walk to the door to get groceries, so I stayed inside all the time and ordered food online. I never knew it was so easy to stay in bed all the time and still get the things I needed to sustain my life. I was miserable for nearly a year.

My dear friend Kate who had been doing CrossFit for nearly ten years, came over one day and told me to get dressed in the most comfortable workout clothes I had. I said I didn't have any workout clothes so I put on a dress and pumps and off we went.

> "It was easier being miserable, so I chose that path until it was too unbearable to be miserable any longer."

I was kicking and screaming but who cared? I was out of the house for the first time since my husband passed, and it felt wonderful and odd at the same time. I knew where she was taking me and I didn't resist too much more because it was for my own good.

When she pulled up in front of a CrossFit place, I was happy to be there, although still anxious because I was not an athlete of any kind. One of my sons who is in the Air Force told me about CrossFit and how he lifts heavy weights and does this and that, and I said hell, no. Inside, I was envious of those people who did CrossFit.

It took me five minutes to get up the courage to get out of her car, but I did and we went inside. As soon as I crossed that threshold, I was again mortified. There were 10 or so very fit people in their 20s and 30s, doing stretches and preparing for the next class. As I watched them, I knew I could never bend over like that so I started to turn and head back to Kate's car.

She gently grabbed my arm and led me over to meet John, a young man who resembled my son who is in his mind-30s. I felt warm and scared at the same time, and he seemed to understand my apprehension.

We followed him as he walked slowly around the "box" and showed me the various sections. There were stacks of weights and thick ropes that went up to the ceiling twenty feet overhead, and barbells and dumbbells and all sorts of other things I knew I'd never be able to lift.

> "CrossFit WODs produce a different kind of pain: it's exquisite and delicious and I love it more than champagne and oxygen. Okay, maybe not champagne."

I couldn't hear a word John said, because I was too caught up in the horror of knowing I couldn't do any of the things in this gym. What the hell was I doing here!?

John stopped his presentation and led me over to a group of four women who were stretching and bending. He introduced me to them and they immediately took me under their wing and asked me questions and told me about how it was for them at first.

I felt less anxious and soon began to open up a little and offered some stories about my family. To make a long story short, that was two years ago when I was a fraidy cat and about forty pounds overweight, and looking and feeling fat.

Today, I am feeling great, can run three miles at about nine minutes' pace, and I do all the exercises in each of our sessions. I can't tell you how hard it was just to get up and start. It was easier being miserable, so I chose that path until it was too unbearable to be more miserable.

I've never been an athlete but now I call myself one, because I run and jump and move really well, and I discovered that I have excellent hand-eye and foot-eye coordination! The discoveries I've made have changed my life, and I wish I could tell every woman who is now like I used to be. I would tell her that all it takes is *showing up*!

As for my diet, well, I've changed that entirely. I no longer drink wine. I no longer eat donuts for breakfast. I now eat salads and light meals and drink lots of water.

Life is so different when your body is in good shape. I can't imagine what I'd be like if I'd not started CrossFit. It depresses me to think about it.

Bobby T Tells It!

The first time I talked with Bobby T, I thought he was an electron that bounced off every surface close to him. He had high energy, great enthusiasm for life, and was pleased to chat about it all.

Bobby T shares his story:

I was one of those high school athletes who was good at that level but not good enough for college sports. In the 1970s, I played football and lifted weights like most guys, but I never really enjoyed any of it. My brothers pushed me into it so I went along.

After high school I got a job in construction and did that for twenty-five years, and it nearly killed me. I fell off a roof onto pavement and broke a few of my vertebrae near my lower back, my lumbar region. It took me ten years to recover, but by the time my back was healed, I was fat. And I mean really fat, like 300 pounds fat.

"CrossFit was a bitch in the beginning. I couldn't even pick up the men's 45-lb. barbell to do a clean, jerk or snatch. Pathetic. I wanted to quit every freakin day but no one would let me."

The first thing I did after a doctor visit was to go home and cry like a little kid. I was so sad about everything. I'd been on some kind of welfare for almost ten years, because my disability ran out, and was left with pretty much nothing. I lost my house that I'd bought at twenty, and that nearly killed my spirit.

After seeing the number on the scales, something inside me changed right then. My doctor said I was high in just about everything, like cholesterol, triglycerides, blood pressure. He said the first thing I needed to do was change what I was eating and drinking.

I loved Dr Pepper! And Little Debbie treats. And ice cream! No wonder I was so fat and unhappy and a wreck of a man. I was pathetic.

One thing kept me going, though. That number on the scale at my doctor's office: 297 lbs. I knew it was bad but I ignored it and all the warning signs of an early death. And I was drinking beer and doing cigarettes too. It was a waste of a life.

My doctor helped me plan my exercise each month. He said we'd start out with eating less, and drinking only water or water with a little fruit flavoring. That was the first three months of my transformation. I went in after 90 days and had lost 27 pounds!

Next he had me do intermittent fasting with vegetable and fruit juice I made myself. I bought this Breville juicer I'd seen on a movie, *Fat, Sick and Nearly Dead*. It was also a life-saver for me.

Skipping to my 55th birthday, I had gotten down to 190 lbs. but that wasn't just fat. I had built up some solid muscle from this new exercise I started. CrossFit! I've now done it for five years and I got to tell you it made me a whole different man. I don't recognize myself in pictures anymore. That wasn't me. And I have such large amounts of energy that I run around like a little kid.

CrossFit was a bitch in the beginning. I couldn't even pick up the men's 45-lb. barbell to do a clean, jerk or snatch. Pathetic. I wanted to quit every freakin day but no one would let me.

I had this sign made that said 297 on it. Nothing too embarrassing. Just the number. Everyone knew what it meant, and they would go to the lockers on top and grab it when I tried to quit. I cried in front of a bunch of guys and they let me cry. Some put their arms around me and said to hang in there. Others held up the sign and patted my back.

They did that a lot the first year, lemme tell you.

It took me two years to get into decent shape to do CrossFit, but I stuck with it. People at the box told me the same stuff. I need to not think about doing the work. Just show up and do it without thinking about it.

Just show up, Bobby. You can do this. You got this, Bobby!

If you listen to good people long enough, their words stick in your brain and you don't just listen to them, you do what they tell you.

That is what I call progress!

As of April 2021, I am 180 pounds of lean muscle, and I have a great attitude to go with it. I teach Bootcamp to newbies who aren't ready for CrossFit, and I share my story with them all the time.

I still have that sign that says 297, and I show it to people once in a while. I like to bring it out after I squat 400 pounds or clean 225. I'm not the strongest in the box, but I am an animal some days.

Best of all, I am different from anything I could have imagined. I eat good food, drink lots of water, and try to sleep at least eight hours a night. I'm now 63, but my genes have me looking about 45, tops.

My skin isn't stretched out like a lot of other men my age, and I feel so much better. Tell you the truth, I don't remember how bad I was back then. I only know how I feel now.

Fan[BLEEPING]tastic!

My Turn Now.

Like many others, my CrossFit journey began when I was at a really low point in my life: overweight and in bad shape from injuries in the Army and from civilian special-operations work I did overseas.

It took many years for me to realize that life doesn't always turn out the way you want. Mine had been a grand life, but there was much pain and anguish in there, too. So much so that I felt so unbelievably tired and worn down all the time.

Feeling awful isn't what I wanted so, after many years of abusing alcohol and cigarettes and not exercising or eating properly, I finally gave up the abuse and started down that road to good health.

We live in a fast-food world that promises us riches and delivers garbage. We succumb to the thousands of advertisements and announcements and enticements each day, and end up depressed and disconnected. The horrible design of our adult lives was planned this way by people who don't care about us except that we open our bank account for them so they can take our money.

"Since starting CrossFit, I've been eating much less but I still do the refined sugars far too much. Just habit that is very hard to break. It was easy to stop drinking alcohol and smoking cigarettes."

Costly cable tv, usurious credit cards, pricey shoes and clothes, the list is seemingly endless. I fell into the very disrepair they wanted me to, and I freely gave them my money.

At some point when I had just turned 58, I didn't make any resolutions or promises. I did what the other people in this story did: *I showed up*. And I kept showing up each day.

I showed up for work without having drunk any alcohol the night before.

I showed up home later that night without having smoked any cigarettes that day.

I showed up in my kitchen and prepared my first juice.

And I kept showing up.

Soon, too, I was standing in a big CrossFit box, talking with a couple owners who gave me their pitch about the benefits of CrossFit. They did tell me I wasn't ready for CrossFit but that I should try their Bootcamp instead.

I agreed and did that for six months. The feeling was uplifting. I now had a strong sense of well-being. My moods were positive. My dreams were pleasant again. But it still wasn't what I needed in the long run.

I was missing out on the benefits from lifting heavy weights in many different styles and positions. I knew I was depriving myself of perhaps the most beneficial part of CrossFit: Olympic-style weightlifting.

Soon as I felt decent, I changed gyms and started doing actual CrossFit. My muscles were sore but I could move in a different way. I wasn't as tight when getting out of bed.

I could sleep an entire eight hours each night without waking up in pain. I could enjoy getting up each morning and looking forward to the day.

It was an unexpected transformation and I loved every bit of it, though it was painful at times, both mentally and physically. But the cool thing was that I kept doing it each week.

I'd love to tell you I do CrossFit seven days a week. I don't. Three times a week, including a private session(s), is good for me, plus the yoga I do at home.

I'm not a yoga person who goes to those big rooms with thirty women and two men, and follows someone else's stretching routine. Boring to me.

> Running on an AirRunner is like running on air. No kidding. And it builds up your hamstrings, calf muscles and soleus unlike any other mechanical exercise device.

I do it in the comfort of my own home, with the music I choose to rock out to or nearly fall asleep to.

I have plenty of yoga bolsters and other supporting tools and a few comfortable mats and wide rubber knee pads for comfort.

Forgot to tell you: I know many people do not like machines like the stationary bike and treadmill, but I need you to take a listen here: I invested $5,000 in an Assault AirRunner and AirBikeElite. Best investments I've made in years.

This just in: Assault was issued a cease-and-desist order by the company that owns the patents on a non-motorized treadmill. It remains to be seen if the AirRunner will remain on the open market. Still, I am forever grateful that I bought mine and use it every day.

The AirRunner is a non-motorized treadmill that burns 30% more calories than a traditional motorized treadmill. Because it is sloped upward in front of you, it works the back of your legs in ways no other machine can. The only other exercise that mimics this movement is running uphill on a slight incline.

The AirRunner also has a heavy-duty belt you run on. Combined with the incline, it encourages you to run naturally like you would run barefoot outdoors, i.e. on the front third of your foot. This style of running is much better for you because it spares the knees and hips from too much trauma over time.

Running on the front third of a foot employs your long spring ligament (your arch), which is largely not used with heel-strike running. The ligament is designed to flex when the front third of a foot hits the ground, store potential energy during this flexion, and then release the energy by springing back and propelling the foot forward.

When you run heel-first, the shock is absorbed in the heel bone, knee joint and hip joint. After years, it kills your joints and works its way up to your lower back, then later your upper back and shoulders.

Running on an AirRunner is like running on air. No kidding. And it builds up your hamstrings, calf muscles and soleus unlike any other mechanical exercise device. Outside of running up a hill many times, the AirRunner builds and strengthens the back of your legs, while also working the quadriceps in front, depending on how high you lift your legs each stride and how far forward you extend each foot.

What I've discovered so amazing, you must try it: my calves, soleus and hamstrings have not looked and felt this good in decades. For my AirRunner workouts, I do modified tabatas: six total minutes of fast-walking, punctuated by three, twenty-second sprints where I extend my feet much farther and thus run much faster than normal. In those 20 seconds, I do at least 100 foot-strikes.

I could never perform this workout on the street. No way. While there are those who say it's not the same as running on the street, I agree with them. I also say that I don't care to run on a street or outdoor hard surface ever again. Don't need to unless running from a hurricane or tornado. Or maybe a crocodile.

Same is true for the AirBikeElite: the heavily padded seat and hand grips make for an ultra-comfortable ride. I ride the bike after doing the AirRunner, but only for two minutes, with four really fast and hard 30-second sprints throughout.

Combined with the AirRunner, the rewards from riding the bike are numerous: big fat burn because of the anaerobic sprints, increased muscle tone and mass, strengthened tendons and ligaments.

I get deep-tissue massages every week, and I love dropping a hundred bucks on my own health and well-being. It's a luxury for me, one I value very much. I'm not suggesting that everyone do this; just wanted to point out the benefits. Fact is, none of us could afford all the extra recovery aids that worldclass athletes use. It would cost us $10,000 a month!

In case you might be wondering, the massage-therapy sessions tease apart the muscle fibers and overlying connective tissue, allowing a better and faster recovery. Sometimes, too, an 800-mg tablet of Ibuprofen does the trick, and that's practically free.

Diet and nutrition? While I address this in detail in Chapter 11, I share a bit here. I used to eat a lot at one sitting. Since I was heavily involved in outdoor activities that severely taxed my body, I needed 6,000 calories at a time. Thing is, as I grew older and less active, especially from injuries, I didn't need those extra calories so they became stored fat and I gained unneeded weight, about fifty pounds.

Since starting CrossFit, I've been eating less but I still do the refined sugars far too much. Just a bad habit that is very hard to break, mostly because I'm fighting trillions of very smart and ruthless microbes in my gut.

Thank goodness it was easy to stop drinking alcohol and smoking cigarettes. I simply changed the way I thot about both. Used to love that burn at the back of throat, esp. with lotsa beer. Changed that thot to hating the smell of it, knowing its 4,000+ chemicals were nothing but harmful to me, it costs a lot of money every month, it was killing me slowly, it was the dumbest thing I was doing.

Quitting drinking was easy. Previously for more than 40 years, I loved that two-beer buzz I got and tried desperately to maintain over many hours of partying. I always ignored and dismissed whatever happened afterward, usually a bad hangover and loss of 48 hours because of it.

For the next two days or so I was basically worthless after 6-12 beers. So I changed my thinking: beer is expensive, bloats me, costs a lot of money every month, makes me fat, makes me dull headed after many, is killing my liver slowly and killing me at the same time.

But to stop eating sugars is still a challenge. That's because of all those trillions of little bacteria and other microbes in my GI tract, telling me to feed them sugar sugar sugar!

The most thing, too, was deciding that I would *exercise* and not train. Huge difference! When I used to train in the military, it was 24/7/365. I couldn't possibly maintain that high operational tempo all my life. Besides, it's more fun to slow down, take a deep breath, exercise and enjoy the whole process.

My wish for you is that you discover the new healthy, fit and beautiful person in you.

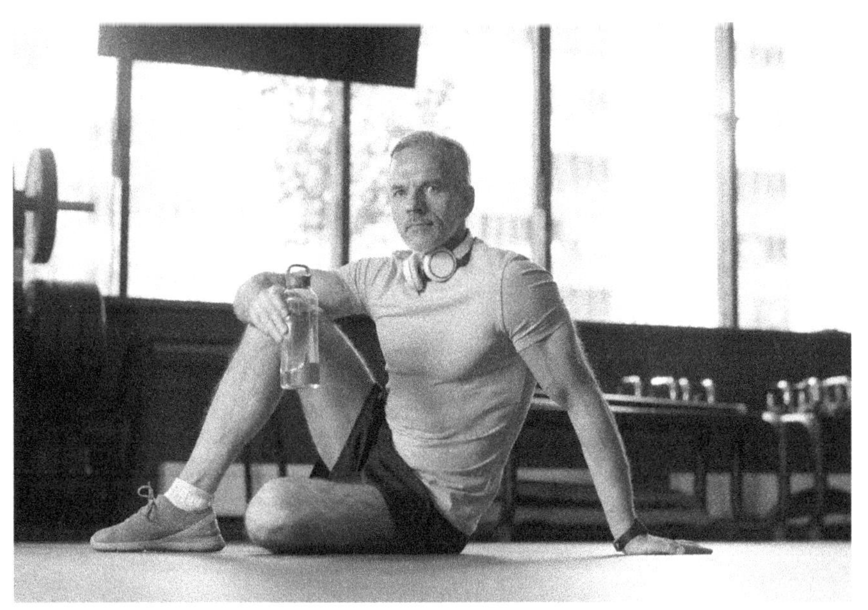

11

Diet, Nutrition and Exercise

"Your eating habits are determined by a hundred trillion little creatures you cannot see."

—Chris Winter

Like it or not, you can't possibly be the best version of you. And we can never know what that version is because there isn't enough time to analyze everything in enough detail. Once you understand and respect these facts, you can focus on living in the moment, day to day, and accepting that what you are today is the "best of you." For now.

As I stated previously, if you took all the advice from experts in CrossFit, weightlifting, yoga, nutrition, etc. you would need 250 hours in each day to fulfill those suggestions from those "experts. What society tells us is far from what we should be doing on our own, but we are stripped of our personal power by a controlling mechanism that we allow to invade our lives every day.

Without our own personal guidance, how can we possibly become the best version of us? No one knows you better than you know you, but we've all been taught to ignore our own feelings and thoughts, and to adopt those of so-called experts.

A giant pile of crap, I say.

Advertisements blast us every day from all forms of media, telling us we can be better if we just do this, do that, and do it all now:

Pay just $99.99 and get *these* benefits. [Gotcha.]

Get on our monthly plan for just $149.95 and you'll become the best you ever. [Uh-huh.]

Come join us at Camp Cure Anything for only $599, and we will transform you into an unrecognizable you. [Right.]

Over the years, I've fallen victim to those scams and discovered an important fact: they promise the moon and the stars but deliver something far less appealing. Those were the days when I was desperate to make a significant change, like quitting alcohol.

Little did I know, I was just too lazy to do the right thing: change my way of thinking about alcohol. Or cigarettes. Or food. My values were all wrong and the consequences were dire.

You Truly Become What You Eat

When I was growing up in Europe in the '60s and '70s, my parents pretty much told me what to eat, and they also allowed me to choose what I wanted when we dined out. That's when, living in Italy, I discovered the miracle of the 7-course dinner.

Italy isn't just some destination, it is a way of life for many who choose it. I was fortunate to have been born into an Air Force family that gave me the gift of travel and lots of it. We visited dozens of countries and learned the people, language, culture, cuisine and how to fit in and learn from the inside.

I loved the food in Italy, especially the fifth course of my favorite meal at Orsini's: canneloni in a rich white sauce with cheese. It would later become my comfort food, although I never mastered the recipe like Signore Orsini.

When we consume rich foods like pasta and cream sauce, certain microbes in our gut become more active and flourish. These are the bad bacteria and associated yeasts and—who knows?—some other unidentified organisms.

Unfortunately, they tell your brain to feed them more of the same and, after decades, you slowly develop diabetes and colon cancer and other terribles. I know 'cos I got one or two of those little shits, and it was because a demon voice inside me was ordering me to do things I didn't wanna do. That voice is actually the collective brain of a trillion little microbes in my gut.

It's not that the Italians have short lives—they most certainly do not. Fact is, they live to be 100 more often than we do. So how is it their rich food, when consumed each day or week, is killing Americans?

Under the cloak of anonymity, one Italian chef told me that Americans demand rich, heavy creams, sauces and desserts. Italians don't consume the "Italian food" we Americans eat, she said. When she feeds her family, they adhere strictly to a healthful Mediterranean diet, rich in fish, nuts, greens, and extra-virgin olive oil. They avoid sugars and they do not consume a lot of red meat.

That same chef told me that almost all countries feed America what it craves: heavy, high-caloric, buttery, cheesy, sugary food. It wasn't always this way. Only in the past 50+ years have things changed for the worse, with the advent of the fast food culture. All those bad bacteria and fungi inside our gut suddenly came alive!

So now the secret was out: the world feeds America delicious foods rich in hydrogenated fat like heavy creams and butter, and too much salt and sugary products. These rich meals, sauces and desserts are addictive and keep us coming back for more. In effect, because of our cravings we are slowly getting fatter and less healthy, and moving to an early grave, thanks to the bad gut microbes that have hijacked our body.

Everything In Moderation, Even Poisons

Did you know it's possible to consume some poisons for years, long as they're taken in moderation?

It's true: we do it every day when we eat processed food like chips, cookies, candy, prepared meals, ice cream, white bread, etc. All the nutrition has been chemically removed from them. Those food companies then add "vitamins" and whatnot so it appears they are serving us a healthful meal.

We don't see these as poison because we've been programmed not to. They tell us all these poisonous foods are good for us because they're delicious and they contain Vitamin C and niacin (and other stuff in laughably insignificant concentrations).

The millions of advertisements teach us to consume junk food and it works well. Just look at the statistics: fast-food companies, processed-food giants, and soft-drink companies all earn billions of dollars each year, peddling the worst nutrition anywhere.

Somehow, we succumb to the temptation and buy hundreds of dollars' worth each year. That cheeseburger and fries you just ate for lunch? Its harmful ingredients are now a part of you, with only a small fraction of them being eliminated from your beautiful body.

The trans fats we see in most of those foods come in two varieties: natural and artificial. The natural fats come from meat and dairy products. Artificial fats are produced on an industrial scale by combining hydrogen with vegetable oil to increase the viscosity—make it more like a stable solid.

Those artificial fats are hard on your body: they contribute to increasing the level of your bad cholesterol and decreasing your good cholesterol (HDL), which leads to hardening and clogging of your arteries.

The effects of junk food and empty-calorie drinks are so numerous, it would take hundreds of pages to explain. What's worse, organizations like the American Heart Association (AMA) do not actually tell us to stop consuming these harmful foods. The AMA soft-pedals the issue by saying we should "reduce consumption of trans fats."

Here's what I say: don't consume any fast foods or processed foods or junk drinks at all. Stay away from processed sugar like high-fructose corn syrup. All are killing America slowly and the AMA is practically encouraging it.

Simple as that. On paper, at least. As you now know, I am still struggling with this issue, though I consume much less junk than before, thanks in no small part to exercising.

Yes, I did say it's possible to consume poisons in moderation, but I was being ironic and silly. It was an example of the resilience of our body in the face of a bad diet. It is possible to consume garbage for years or decades, cease putting that crap in your body, then allow it to heal through good diet and exercise.

I've done experiments on myself over the years, changing my diet and trying new things, though admittedly I still do battle with those bad microbes in my gut that demand a pint of Jamoca Almond Fudge ice cream and a few double-cheeseburgers.

"Mind over matter" is a difficult concept to implement when you're fighting a shadowy enemy that wants you to feed it sugar sugar sugar. That enemy is made up of more than 100 trillion microbes that have a huge say in what you eat and how often, and how you feel in general.

Though you may not believe it, those microbes have a collective mind of their own and they are experts at hijacking your beautiful mind. We are only just beginning to understand how our own gut microbes do what they do, and learning how to counter some of their behaviors so we don't fall into disrepair.

More on that in Chapter 12.

About Your Diet

You've read countless books, articles, posts, etc. on the importance of adopting and maintaining proper balanced nutrition. I will not insult your intelligence or wealth of knowledge here. What I do wanna share with you are the simple facts we now know and understand about a good healthful diet.

As I shared with you earlier, I still struggle like a madman about adopting a good diet for me. It's an uphill battle every single day and I'm fighting that invisible enemy: my own gut microbes. This has been going on all my life, my eating both good foods and unhealthful crap. In doing so, I've built a resident population of bad microbes in my gut and they now boss me around like I was an obedient child.

Consciously I strive not to eat sugars and other junk, and I've been successful in cutting back significantly. But not stopping altogether like I did alcohol and cigarettes. It seems my gut microbes didn't care much whether I drank and smoked, so I could quit cold turkey without much fuss.

Food, on the other hand, is a whole different beast. Something tells me I will be battling my gut microbes well into the future. In the least, though, I am learning much more about my own chemistry and behavior, cravings and how and when they appear, and how to slowly change my diet for the better.

Enough of me. Let's chat about diet, in general, and how it affects exercise.

Every person is different. We understand this. What we don't seem to get is the fact that all those books on diet and exercise are speaking only generally and sometimes do not apply to you. They offer fad diets of all stripe and, if you study them over the decades, you discover that they come and go so quickly we forget all about them.

There are some generalizations we can make about how diet influences our level and quality of exercise. Some things are just plain bad for you and everyone else. Some things are good for everyone, as well.

When a diet calls for "protein," what is it really saying? There're many types of protein and, in the end, it is the amino acids we need.

Carbohydrates come in all varieties, too. Our tissues and cells need carbs but exactly what kind? Those that're not processed: natural high-carb foods like potatoes and carrots and quinoa.

Fats? America was ambushed in the 1950s when Dr. Ancel Keys suggested we avoid fats because they caused heart disease. He's the guy after whom WWII K-rations were named, because he developed the recipes (yes, he told me so). He's also the man who conducted the first human starvation experiments (on conscientious objectors during WWII).

I read both volumes of his books, *Human Starvation*, and talked and corresponded with him about my own five-month-long "starvation experiment," where I lost 50 pounds of mostly muscle (long story there, not safe for work).

Since Dr. Keys' pronouncement almost 70 years ago, fats have been the bad guy, something to avoid altogether. The truth is that our cells need certain types of fats, or fatty acids or triglycerides. We synthesize our own fats from the food we eat.

Essential fats like Omega-3 fats (in fish and flax seed) and Omega-6 fats (in nuts, seeds and vegetable oil) must be included in your diet.

The issue with so-called fats is simple: the food industry has flooded the market with unhealthful fats in the form of trans fats, which are artificial, industrially produced fats that prolong shelf life and can be used over and over in cooking.

We do have a good idea what the general ratio of proteins, carbohydrates and fats should be in our diet: about 1/3 protein, less than 2/3 carbos (much of those in the form of prebiotics to feed and nurture the gut microbes), and a small amount of natural healthful fats.

What people forget to consider are the other ingredients of a healthful diet: natural vitamins (not supplements), minerals (essential and trace), prebiotics, probiotics, intermittent fasting, water, and air (esp. oxygen and carbon dioxide).

There are dozens of different methods of fasting and I've tried several. If you want to lose weight fast and "reset" your metabolism, so to speak, do a one-week juice diet. I process a gallon of fruit/vegetable juice from 20 lbs. of fruits and vegetables, using a Breville juicer, and dilute it 50% with distilled water.

Unfortunately, this diet is not sustainable over the long run. For me, I do it twice a year and feel refreshed after each week.

I've tried many different pill and powder supplements over 30-plus years, using my 6-months-on, 6-months-off regimen. It allows any given drug to take effect so I can note its efficacy.

The only supplements that made any discernible difference in my behavior, health, well-being, blood/urine chemistry were vitamin C, sodium bicarbonate and nicotine (patch).

Currently, I make a fresh drink of liquid vitamin C and sodium bicarbonate powder in distilled water. Usually I drink a glass after CrossFit and feel less sore and more energetic. Since I've experimented with this drink for many years, I know the positive effects are real.

A short word on nicotine: it is not addictive. I won't argue that point with anyone. It is non-addictive. Period. I use it as a cognitive enhancer, something to boost my thinking and awareness. Not every day, though. It's a bit too much for me.

Honestly, I prefer my current state of "medium-level thinking" and "good" awareness, rather than a heightened state of each. Did you ever see that movie *Limitless*? Taking nicotine (21 mg/day) is like being max-wired like Bradley Cooper's character. Sure, I got more work done in a shorter time because I was focused on each task and not distracted by anything else, but I felt like a robot going 100 mph all day.

Oh, forgot to mention: there is a price to pay for revving up your metabolism unnaturally by taking supplements like nicotine: eventually you will crash and the rebound can be very unpleasant.

No, thank you! I share this anecdote about nicotine as a gentle warning: be careful what you wish for, because everything comes with side effects and unintended consequences.

Perhaps most bothersome of all: people don't test supplements before taking them. They read up on something or get a recommendation from a doctor, family member or friend, and then they blindly ingest it. Worse, still, is the sad fact that people will take a dozen different supplements at once. Even several times a day.

How do you know whether a supplement benefits you? Or whether it harms you, especially in the long run? How do you tease apart the individual effects? It's impossible to answers these questions when you take multiple supplements at once.

What most don't consider: the efficacy of each supplement confounds the performance of all the others, so you cannot say which one is actually beneficial and which is/are detrimental to your health and well-being.

Very few people realize that you must get a baseline blood and urine analysis done so you know your general health. Then you must take the time to test each supplement, one by one, over a long-enough period time for the drug to rise to an efficacious concentration in the body. And then you must take good notes each day about how you feel and perform, and do this trial over six months. At least.

And if you wanna be really thorough, do what I've done for decades: repeat each experiment at least one more time to see if you get the same results. After doing this for more than 30 years, I finally decided on what worked for me and what was a complete waste of money, time, effort.

Sadly, almost all supplements are made in China and, according to one major supplier in the US, there is no direct quality control of products. American companies simply trust what the overseas labs report to them on quality of products.

My personal feelings about most supplements: dubious short-term gains are not worth jeopardizing my long-term health. I have enough problems dealing with the trillions of demonic microbes in my gut.

I've written a partial list of "avoids and adds" to get you started. Sure, you've probably heard it all before, but now you need to read them carefully and implement what you learn here and in your other readings.

I know it's easier said than done, because you are battling some bad microbes in your gut, and they have a strong say about what you eat. But it can be done with lotsa patience and practice.

The key is to stick to it, day in and day out, until you hit that special milestone that pushes you over those bad habits. Once you reach it, and you will feel when it happens, you may not return to the old diet again.

Personally, this is my biggest challenge in life: fighting bad microbes that scream for sugar and processed carbs. If I had one wish in life, it would not be about wealth or power. I would wish for a 100% healthy gut and all its "good" inhabitants.

Things to avoid:

Sugar, especially adding them to your meals. Sucrose and high-fructose corn syrup are toxic. Artificial sweeteners are toxic.

Sugary drinks, even sports drinks and energy drinks. Period.

Candy of any kind.

Cereals with any amount of sugar.

Trans fats like those in commercially produced foods.

Processed foods of any kind. Their ingredients include toxic byproducts like stabilizers and colorings and preservatives, plus things we aren't allowed to know about.

Red meat, i.e. beef, lamb, pork, veal. These animal products are often difficult enough to digest. Hidden additives that meat producers need to keep meat looking good on the shelf.

Things to add to your diet:

Leafy green vegetables like lettuce, spinach, kale, Swiss chard, Romaine lettuce, etc.

Carrots, beets, celery, broccoli, tomatoes, cauliflower, mushrooms.

Beans and legumes.

Potatoes, in moderation.

Bananas and most other fruit.

Turkey and chicken, both in moderation. That is, do not eat them every day. I suggest buying the best meats that're certified hormone and antibiotics free. And those grown on animal-friendly farms.

Your Exercise Routine Depends On Proper Nutrition

Face it: when you eat, you are feeding not only yourself. You are feeding trillions of microbes in your gut. Sometimes, you have little to no say over what you consume. Yes, that is an absolute fact. I can tell you this from my own personal experience. It's like having a demon inside you.

If you're like me, struggling with adopting and maintaining a proper diet, please re-read this section. Read it again. And again. I've kept it simple enough so I don't overwhelm you. Or myself. Yup, I read it over and over, too. A little of it sticks each time.

While you do not have to have a great diet before you start CrossFit, I suggest you find a good nutritionist to assist you in starting one. You'll find it easier to engage in CrossFit, and you'll enjoy yourself much more because you will feel great before, during and after workouts. And your body will heal faster so you can continue.

When you begin a workout, you initially start with an oxygen deficit. That means that your muscles do not have adequate oxygen to power them. This anaerobic phase dissipates as you warm up and then do hard-core CrossFit exercises. It can ramp up again if you do high-intensity work that depletes oxygen in muscles.

Initially, that oxygen comes from the air you breathe. It binds to hemoglobin and later myoglobin in the muscles, where it releases oxygen from capillaries to muscle cells and larger fibers. Those muscles cells must also have a continuous source of the energy molecule called ATP (adenosine triphosphate).

Under exercise work, it undergoes transformation from ATP to ADP (adenosine diphosphate) and back to ATP again. The bonds that are broken release a lot of energy used by our mitochondria to power each cell.

Interestingly, our mitochondria were engineered into our cells. Previously, on the evolutionary scale, they had been independent bacteria, probably not too unlike the bacteria in your gut. So it's not a stretch to believe that the bacteria in our gut are very important to our overall health and well-being.

Interestingly, too, mitochondria also have their own DNA (mitochondrial DNA or mDNA) that's propagated down the genetic line by *females.*

When you do CrossFit, you're recruiting more of your muscles in each muscle group to perform an exercise. And when you do high-intensity work, you not only recruit more muscles, you push them to work much harder than they have ever worked before.

The result is that your muscles can withstand harder workouts for a longer period of time. You endurance goes way up. This is important to you in everyday life, because you now can do all those household chores without panting, without muscles aches and pains, and with more fluidity and flexibility.

All things considered, your working muscles during CrossFit primarily require oxygen and energy, and they get it from proper breathing and a good diet. Trust me here: if your diet is inadequate, you will feel fatigued and tired, your muscles will be sore and will not heal quickly, and you will experience an overall lethargy that saps your strength.

You may also feel depressed and anxious, and your head will be foggy, like it's filled with cotton. Not a good feeling, is it? And to think it's primary due to your unhealthful diet, something you have the power to change.

Now onto the hardest chapter of all, something I've avoided for a long time. Gotta admit, though, it's the most fascinating subject I've ever studied in my life.

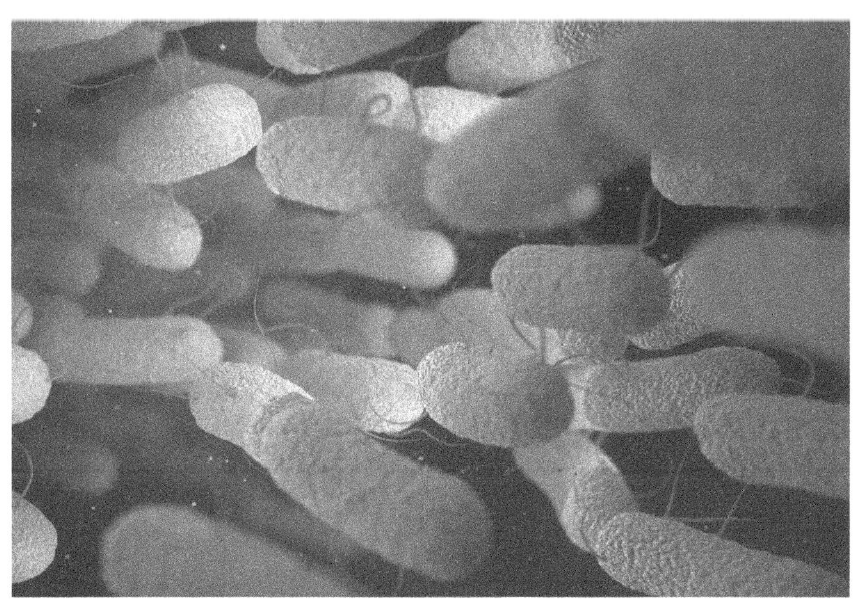

12

Your Gut Microbes and Exercise

"Your gut microbes form a new superorgan and organ system that influences, manipulates and controls your chemistry and behavior."
—Chris Winter

Disclaimer: In the interest of fairness and accuracy, I'm letting you know that some of the information in this chapter is based on my hypotheses and not on 100% proven facts. In turn, I base these informed and educated ideas on sound scientific and medical facts I've gathered and analyzed. It's my feeling they will be proven accurate in the coming years.

Over time I've discovered that it's best to learn about a subject by bingeing on as much available information as possible. My subconscious needed to consume it all at once and distill it down to its essence. Chapter 13 details the human subconscious, how it works and how to make it work for you.

In using this binge approach I was able to see unique patterns of information that others missed, did not consider, or have yet to discover. Since I am no longer a scientist and have no boss to answer to, I can get away with discussing fringe ideas and share with you my deep thoughts that I know are accurate and true. They just haven't been recognized by the mainstream scientific and medical establishment. Yet.

Though working scientists will likely dismiss my ideas, I pray you will not only consider them but also dive deep into this fascinating subject. You don't have to be formally trained in science or medicine to read a paper on this subject, do your own research, and perhaps discover something new and important.

There's a growing field of "amateur" scientists, i.e. those without PhDs and MDs, who experiment with gene editing and produce fascinating and relevant results, so who's to say you can't do good experimental science that benefits you and many others?

Sometimes It's Best To Do Things On Your Own

For several weeks in May 2021, I agonized over a subject I had been studying intensively for many months. My subconscious told me it was probably the most important organ system in the human body, influencing all other organs and organ systems and in ways well beyond the imagination.

Science was only beginning to study its wide-ranging effects, but no one laboratory or person had yet defined it, much less described how it all worked.

Sometimes those we rely on for answers have no idea what they're studying, nor can they explain it to the rest of us so we can understand it and benefit from it. And sometimes key data and results are withheld from us for whatever reasons.

That's when I get frustrated because I want answers to all my questions about how my body works and what I can do to change things for the better. Try as I do, I've still not figured out how best to heal my gut, which I know is contributing to my overall health.

Like others, for decades I've sensed that what I ate had a profound effect on my actions, behaviors, moods, emotions, and cognitive state. And I tried many different "therapies" to heal myself. Thing is, I never knew what was actually inside my gut that may have acted against me.

Until now. I finally found a reputable lab that analyzes at least a portion of the gut microbiome from fecal samples. I hate to be chatting on with you about my personal poo, but there ya go. As I explain at the end of this chapter, the results and recommendations based on analysis of my own gut microbes have given me a new path to consider on my way to better health.

I suggest you do an online search for "gut health test" or "gut microbes test." Since this field is new, it's considered the wild west, with some labs most likely being fly-by-night operations that yield false results.

I wish I could tell you the best labs to try but I'm in the dark, too. I'm simply trying different ones every couple of months, and comparing results, kinda like I did when I had my DNA analyzed by many different labs. The results at times were amusing, to say the least, which is why I say the state of the art of gut microbiome analysis is the wild west.

Still, it's a starting point, one I lacked when trying prebiotics and probiotics years ago. How can you feed the demon inside your gut when you don't even know what food it prefers? It's like feeding a cat bird food: after a day or two, you have one unhappy cat.

My gut microbes also felt the same when I fed them the wrong stuff. Now armed with a general idea of the microbes inside my gut, I can experiment with different foods to see how my gut reacts. It's an ongoing experiment. I pray you will start your own, as well.

The Answers You Seek Are Inside You

In times like these, in the absence of answers from the scientific community, I dive headfirst into the subject and begin my own investigation. I've done that with many different things in my life, and have figured them out well enough to make significant changes in my thoughts, actions, behaviors and how I live.

Since I'd been a scientist years ago, I knew how to start this new journey and what to look for. I began with the existing scientific literature on the subject of the human gut microbial community.

After reading hundreds of books, scientific papers and articles over three months, I soon realized no one had hypothesized the overall role of our gut microbes, nor had they extended it to exercise.

Before moving further, I needed to get a sense of the creatures I was dealing with. For the most part, they were less than a quarter the diameter of a red blood cell, too small for me to see.

They had no eyes I could peer into. No ears to speak to. No mouth to communicate with. No hand to shake in greeting. No traditional form of communicating with this thing.

Undeterred, I lay down with some soothing adagios in the background, closed my eyes, and let my subconscious do the thinking. The next morning when I awakened with a revelation.

When I define something, I start with known characteristics, usually the obvious physical ones. Human gut microbiota act as a diffuse, intelligent swarm. A small sea of intelligent creatures that influence us in untold ways. That much I knew.

Kahuni: Born Of The Sea

I then dived deeper into this "sea" and discovered the microbes perform as a series of waves when they act on the human body. Since I'd switched music from adagios to Bruno Mars, I was struck by his Hawaiian heritage and followed the thought in that direction.

Sea . . .

Wave . . .

Intelligent being . . .

Hawaii . . .

The Hawaiian term *kahuna* means "wise one" . . .

In surfing terms, it means "big wave" . . .

But these little buggers weren't just one being, so I pluralized kahuna to "kahuni."

Laugh if you must, but it fits. It's also that kind of neologism that sticks in your mind. Think: Google, Yahoo, Hulu, etc. It is also a surname of people from Zimbabwe. They're cheering me on right now. Join in at any time.

I came up with the term *kahuni* when thinking about what the microbes inside really are: a sea of very intelligent, living things that influence us and our actions and behaviors, modulate our general chemistry and neurochemistry, and mediate our general health and well-being. This limited definition surely will expand as we learn more.

Only the brain is more diverse in duties and responsibilities, and it now appears that it is also influenced by the kahuni. I wish I could write everything I've learned about this magnificent superorgan, but it is beyond the range of this book.

The kahuni system has unique actions: it acts like an immune system. It also acts like a brain, a central processing unit that affects all organ systems in human body. The kahuni is the body's second brain and its functions and influences are just being revealed.

The kahuni inside us are older than we are, and has been engineered into us to navigate the world of plants and other non-digestible species by acting as a middleman between human and food/stimulus source.

The kahuni is your ambassador to the outside world.

And your kahuni is your adjunct brain and controls more of you than you realize.

Kahuni Nomenclature

To examine the kahuni, we need a new system of names, terms and definitions. Here's a start:

Prokahuni: the good microbes and their associated metabolites and byproducts that support your good health.

Malkahuni = bad microbes that cause health issues and keep you unhealthy.

Pathokahuni = disease-causing microbes.

Kahuniology = the study of the complex biophysical, chemical, ecological, etc. aspects of the human microbiome and its relationship with all other human organ systems, organs, tissues, cells, organelles, DNA, etc.

Kahuniome = the entire set of microbes within the human body.

Kahuniomics = the systematic study of the microbes inhabiting the human body.

Doubtless there will be more as we learn about the specifics of the kahuni and its attendant influences, duties and responsibilities.

Kahuni: What We Know Now

This new subject deserves an entire book, but I'll focus only on a few highlights to give you an idea how the kahuni ecosystem functions inside your body.

The new scientific discipline that studies our gut microbiome is so new that it doesn't have a formal name. As stated earlier, let's remedy that: Kahuniology.

Beyond the name, scientists have examined the kahuni in some detail and come up with a general outline for its various functions. There are now more than 300 new private laboratories around the world, raising millions to study the kahuni. Like testing labs, this is the wild west of modern science and it's likely to continue like this for the next decade and beyond.

These labs are developing drugs and other pharmaceuticals to "cure" the diseases caused by these microbes. They should be studying how to modify and heal our kahuni, which will turn us into healthy beings. Unfortunately, you know the pharmaceutical industry is out to make money by keeping us sick without dying anytime soon.

What's worst of all is the fact that this new industry's lobbyists will eventually write the position papers that become federal laws, forbidding us citizens from studying our own kahuni and learning how to modify it ourselves. They don't want you to know how to heal your body and keep it healthy.

This same legal strategy is being used to keep those "amateur" scientists from studying and modifying the human genome. I believe the kahuni is the key to most if not all diseases in your body, and we should be able to learn about it and change or modify it on our own. We need to learn all we can about our kahuni before we lose the opportunity.

The Big Kahuni Oversees All

It is becoming clear that the kahuni influences or mediates activity in every organ and organ system in the human body. We're also learning that the more diverse the kahuni, the better.

I'm talking about having a wide range of "good" microbes that benefit your health. Those who consume a Western diet seem to have the least-diverse kahuni in the world, and many are the "bad" microbes.

Contrast that with the Mediterranean diet that produces a very healthful and diverse kahuni, with people who not only live to a hundred but they also live well and are generally happier. Those people are not inundated with garbage advertising about junk food like we are in America. Propaganda is alive and well in this country, isn't it?

Here're some examples of how the kahuni interact with you and your body:

The relationship between the kahuni and brain, called the **kahuni-brain axis**, is not known in detail but there are some developments you should pay attention to. Some compounds secreted and excreted by the kahuni diffuse into the bloodstream and directly to the brain where they may influence behaviors like hunger and depression.

Specific kahuni microbes interact with enteroendocrine cells, aka neuropod cells, in the lining of the gut and transmit signals to the brain via the vagus nerve. The result is that kahuni microbes influence certain behaviors in the human host. Yes, bacteria and company are telling you what to do and they're not asking your permission.

There is growing evidence that kahuni may be involved in causing or influencing neurodegenerative diseases like Alzheimer's, Parkinson's, ALS, etc. Imagine that: all these decades we've been looking in all the wrong places. The answer may lie not in the environment, e.g. aluminum or toxins, but inside one's own gut.

The **kahuni-skin axis**: bacteria in the kahuni send out chemicals that cause and modulate acne, skin sensitivity to the sun and chemicals, etc. It also causes dry, itchy skin and is likely responsible for various skin diseases and issues.

The **kahuni-joint axis**: there is some evidence that an imbalance in your kahuni causes osteoarthritis. I hypothesize that it is also responsible for so-called autoimmune diseases like rheumatoid arthritis (RA), systemic lupus erythematosus (lupus), inflammatory bowel disease (IBD) and multiple sclerosis (MS).

Could it be that you can heal yourself from RA simply by adjusting the balance of microbes in your kahuni? If so, what is someone takes away your ability to heal yourself, but instead offers you expensive RA pharmaceuticals that must be taken for the remainder of your life?

Kahuni-digestive system axis: all the microbes in your kahuni are a carbohydrate-fermentation system, breaking down complex carbs that the human gut cells cannot and heavily influencing the amount of available energy inside the colon.

The kahuni also breaks down other complex carbohydrates that the human digestive system cannot. The fermentation process releases energy, vitamins and other compounds that aid in digestion and general health of the human host. The end result is the production of short-chain fatty acids (SCFA) like acetate, butyrate and propionate.

Some prokahuni bacteria in the large intestine produce a short-chain fatty acid, butyrate, from the fermentation of indigestible plant fibers. Butyrate produces 90% or more of the energy for intestinal epithelial cells, and about 15% of the total energy for the human body.

It has a number of important functions in the gut: assists in preventing inflammation and colorectal cancer, and supports the growth of intestinal villi and mucus that lines the gut.

In the absence of a sufficient concentration of butyrate, the intestine becomes inflamed and leaky, thus allowing microbes into the bloodstream where they release endotoxins that cause untold harm in other tissues, organs and organ systems.

The Western diet contributes to decreased numbers of prokahuni that produce butyrate, and thus to diseases resulting from low concentrations of butyrate in the gut.

Acetate is the most abundant SCFA in the gut. It regulates pH, controls hunger and appetite, provides energy to butyrate-producing bacteria, and protects the gut against pathogens.

Again, butyrate provides the energy source for colon cells and helps prevent leaky gut, and protects against inflammation and damage caused by pathogens and their endotoxins.

Propionate acts like butyrate in protecting the gut against inflammation, and like acetate in regulating hunger and appetite.

When we eat junk food, especially containing artificial trans-fats, the general digestive process slows and eventually breaks down and contributes to leaky gut, diarrhea, and even worse issues and diseases.

Your Own Malkahuni Are At War With You

This was the most difficult section for me to write about, and I actively avoided it for months because it's what is killing me slowly: bad nutrition because the nasty microbial community in my gut has only one item on its menu. Sugar.

And my gut microbes apparently have a huge say in how much and how often I must feed them. I'm not ashamed to say, this part of my life absolutely sucks. I hate it. And I hate the fact that trillions of tiny microscopic organisms are bossing me around and keeping me sick, all because they want their sugar fix.

Sadly, I am hosting, maintaining and feeding an entire community of drug addicts who don't care about me. All they want is their hourly fix. And when they don't get it, they jones for more and more, often producing stomach aches and cramps until I shoot 'em up with sugar. They're beyond ungrateful. They are rude.

When you're being hit from all sides, how do you possibly defend yourself? Intellectually, I know what my target is—a trillion tiny torpedoes. Maybe I should just nuke 'em with a wide-spectrum antibiotic. That would cause a lotta collateral damage, though, and I'd be worse off than before. So now what?

I do know that I look pathetic trying to pick out a single target with my BB gun. They overpower me by swarming and acting collectively. Their allied attacks against me easily subjugate my seemingly helpless brain.

Sounds pitiful, doesn't it? Like I said, I'm not embarrassed to share this with you, because I know many of you are also experiencing the same bombardment as I am. Maybe you're thinking the same helpless thoughts? And maybe you're coming up with a good strategy for taking on these little terrors inside your gut.

The short answer is that our Western diet is responsible for the growth of malkahuni that, in turn, are causing untold diseases in us.

Who knows? Maybe we can team up and engage this enemy together. I welcome your thoughts, ideas, suggestions. Meantime, let's chat about what we do know about the link between gut microbial activity and exercise.

The Missing Link: Kahuni And Exercise

It's thought that there are many different species of bacteria and other microbes in our gut, but only certain types are expressed and active at any given time. This depends on the conditions inside your gut, your diet and your level of fitness.

During intense physical activity, prokahuni concentrations increase to produce more energy for other microbes, your own cells in the colon, and for the muscles you're working. These same bacteria and other microbes appear to decrease in concentration when exercises slows or ceases.

Therefore, when you work out, you create a wave of kahuni activity that directly affects your fitness in many ways, e.g. increasing your strength and endurance. Could it be that some prokahuni are turned on and off according to your activity?

We now know that having a diverse megacolony of good microbes in our gut is beneficial to good health, and that being overrun by pathogenic microbes can erode and destroy our intestinal lining, and kill us slowly.

When you are sedentary, some malkahuni are produced in larger concentrations and they cause all manner of health issues and diseases. When you then exercise continually, you effectively keep these malkahuni at bay and promote the growth of prokahuni.

It's possible to manipulate the trillions of resident microbes in your gut and the various metabolites they secrete and excrete. What's more, by doing so, you can also manipulate how these microbes affect your intestinal health.

When you exercise, certain good microbes upregulate their production of certain beneficial amino acids that build proteins. They also turn on other chemical processes that provide more energy to your muscles and support tissues.

Your kahuni are nearly 100% dependent on your diet and whether you take antibiotics. They rely on you to feed them, and in turn they determine what level of fitness you will have, since they are deeply involved in proper functioning of all organs and organ systems. If you take antibiotics, it will disrupt and even destroy many prokahuni, thus causing an imbalance in your gut microbes and level of nutrition.

The Kahuni Is Your Secret Weapon

All the more reason to determine exactly what microbes make up your kahuni via scientific testing. The next step is to feed the good microbes with proper nutrition and avoid all foods that promote the growth of bad microbes.

Given kahuniology is in the infant stage, you will have to experiment on your own what works for you and what does not. Be patient! I know how frustrating it is.

In sum, I hypothesize that your kahuni acts as a mediator with all organs and organ systems, thus providing you a source of energy and protection (via the immune system) during exercise.

It also acts in harmful ways, causing various diseases, ailments and issues that, to date, are thought to be caused by other means, e.g. environmental toxins, food/drink toxins and additives, etc.

Example: psoriasis is a terrible and unsightly skin disease with no cure, or so the medical authorities tell us. I say the answer lies with your kahuni and large intestine, both of which have a large hand in regulating immune and skin functions.

Could it be as simple as a continuously bad diet that feeds harmful microbes in your body and kills off good ones? The doctors I spoke with dismissed me outright and steered me to drugs that treat the symptoms of psoriasis. I immediately dismissed them because I don't take no for an answer and I knew they were ignorant and inexperienced on the subject of the kahuni and how it regulates many processes in the human body.

Also, autoimmune diseases are, in my estimation, caused by an imbalance of microbes and their secretory and excretory byproducts that attack and damage various cells, tissues, organs and organ systems. It's a shame so many people will continue to suffer, though I contend cures are probably associated with our kahuni and could be available to us.

Interestingly, people with one disease or malady tend to have other issues that can be traced back to the kahuni, if only one would take the time to examine things more in depth. There is rarely a disease that has only one focus or target. An imbalance in the kahuni may also be acting on more than one site.

We should be looking for ways to heal a damaged kahuni and learn how to maintain it in good health. Instead, pharmaceutical companies look for drugs that treat the symptoms of these diseases. This suggests we may never know the true function of the kahuni, because the science behind it, and possible cures lying within, will be hidden from us in favor of corporate profits.

By adjusting our own kahuni, we can at least test whether the problems that affect us change for the better or disappear altogether. We may be able to cure ourselves of the various problems that affect us.

Become A Scientist And Physician

It is now up to each of us to study and learn about our own body and kahuni. Each of us is a scientist and physician, and we must act the parts and heal ourselves. This starts with your own self-study and experimentation. Get your kahuni tested by several different laboratories and begin your self-study in earnest.

Funny revelation: after getting back the results of my own gut microbe analysis, I started making a detailed list of all the fruits and vegetables to buy, and an even longer list of those foods I could no longer consume. If I remained true to my new diet. One of the major food recommendations was to completely avoid all potatoes. Seriously.

No more mashed red potatoes, no more hash browns, no more tater tots. And no more potato-couching. All things considered, I am fine with that. Gotta admit, though: I will miss garlicky mashed potatoes. And tater tots. And buttery hash browns. Such are the sacrifices ya gotta make sometimes to be healthy.

Though disappointed in having to eliminate certain foods from my regular diet, I was grateful that I had become my own scientific advisor and personal physician. And I now have the opportunity to test my own kahuni and build a better and more healthful diet. It's the most difficult step of my life, changing what I eat and even more so, fighting that invisible demon inside my own body.

Like I said, I'm a work in progress and I'm now armed with the best tools available at this time. I'm sure I'll discover more in the future. Every week I come across new information about our gut microbes and their relationship to us, and am able to implement some new action in my diet. I imagine the day when my kahuni is balanced and happy, so I can enjoy exercising and improve my health and well-being.

I pray you also become a scientist and physician, and study, analyze, and learn how to heal yourself. What's more, I hope you will maintain that good health throughout your CrossFit journey and your life.

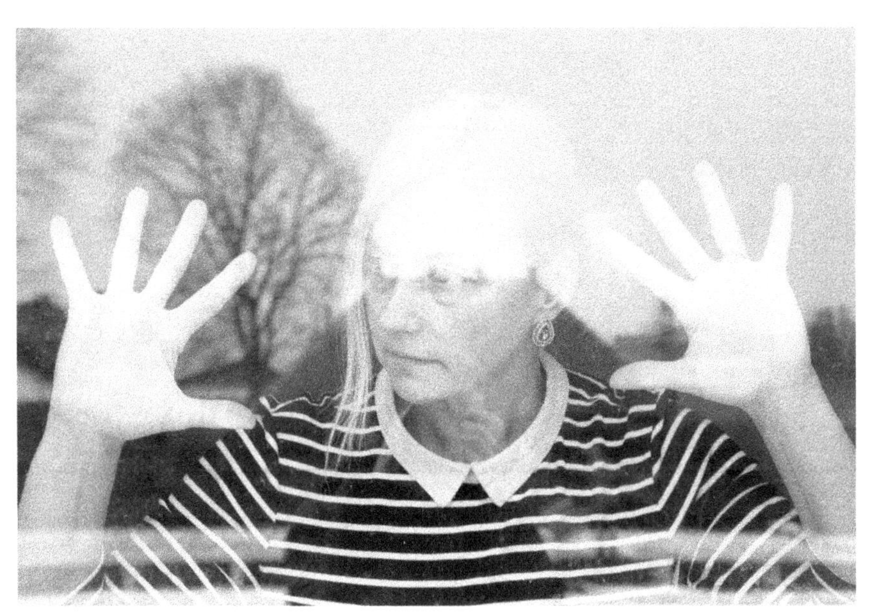

13

Your *Subconscious* Will Guide You to Health and Well-Being

"It doesn't matter whether you believe, because *magic* is all around us."

—Chris Winter

It's time for you to break down the invisible barrier that holds you back and prevents you from knowing the real you. There's a whole universe of magic deep inside you. Like your kahuni, an unchartered expanse filled with the mysteries of space and time.

Since this is fringe information, it is not necessary for your CrossFit journey but I strongly encourage you to give it a try.

They tell us that the last unexplored frontier is outer space or maybe the deep blue sea. Baloney, I say. While it's not the last one, it is certainly the most important in your life right now: your own *subconscious*.

Every waking and sleeping moment your subconscious is hard at work ensuring your safety and security. Most people do not listen to their own subconscious, so it does not work well for them. I am suggesting here that you take a listen to my thoughts on your subconscious, and study it on your own.

You may be pleasantly surprised at what you discover inside yourself and how you can use it in your everyday life.

A Discussion On The Human Subconscious

One of my dear friends who read an early draft of this book suggested I discuss one of my favorite topics: the human subconscious, dreams and dreaming. Many years ago, she and I had long talks about the importance of them in our daily lives.

I showed her what the subconscious was, how it functioned, and the importance of it in dreams and dreaming, and how to use it to fulfill our needs and wants. I asked her how this might be important to someone starting CrossFit.

She didn't hold back: "Are you [dumb] or what, Chris! You taught me that when you harness the power of my subconscious thoughts and actions, something really magical happens. And a new world of possibilities opens up to me.

"I started actively controlling my thoughts when sleeping and, when I did, I could bring new and better things into my life. If you include some of these teachings in your new book, it may open up a world of possibilities for your readers, something far beyond just doing CrossFit.

"And if you yourself would work on it more, you could cure that metabolic disease that's killing you slowly because of your lousy diet."

What would Yoda say?

"Good point, she has. Loves you, she does. Dumb, you are. Listen to her, you should."

I've studied the human subconscious, mostly in myself and a few brave souls, since I was a child, wondering what inner engine drove me to do the things I did. I didn't have to think about doing certain things, I just did them. Sometimes they were rational and positive; other times, not so.

One item I discovered over the years: there was a clear line between how my mind functioned subconsciously and what I did consciously.

And when I went to sleep each night, I knew there was a whole different creature that came alive and took me on endless journeys through space and time, introducing me to new thoughts, ideas, beliefs and ways of doing things in my life.

My CHILD, Finally Discovered

Many years ago, long before CrossFit, I woke up one morning and scrambled out of bed to write something down. Whatever was in my head at that moment had to come out and it wasn't going to wait for my bus driver, my typist, to take dictation.

It was coming in a flood and that was that. When I got to my notepad, my hand started scribbling things down. I wasn't paying attention to what I was writing, I just took it on faith that I had to do this.

After I was done autowriting, I looked at what had emerged: a single word, along with details about each letter of the word. It was an acronym, CHILD:

C: the little Child in you, the curious wide-eyed being who sees the world without filters and preconceived notions about anything. A little sponge that senses things with wonder and awe.

H: the true Heart in you, the purely subjective part, filled with every conceivable emotion. Sees the world smartly but with passion and feeling.

I: your Intuition or information-gathering system, the sensory apparatus that receives every possible stimulus in The Universe, much like a radio receives radio signals to produce spoken word and songs.

L: the cold, stainless-steel Logic that sees the world purely objectively, like a robotic computer that takes in and analyzes data in a totally impartial and neutral way, without emotion or feeling of any kind.

D: the little Demon in you, that mischievous entity that plays pranks and does impish things. Can sometimes be very destructive and hurtful, so it's kept in check by the other entities.

These ethereal beings all comprise the human subconscious, which is the true engine that drives each and every one of us in our daily lives.

They all work together and, depending on how one's DNA is wired, sometimes for good and sometimes for evil. I will not get into the moral implications of good and evil, only stating that they exist in all of us to some extent and, in others, comprise their whole being.

Destiny, Celestiophysics, Subism

We can choose to communicate with our child, or we can ignore it and just float through life, going wherever it takes us. I contend that we do have a destiny.

Each of us, when we are conceived (not born), have a certain imprint from those celestial bodies that mediate and modulate our behaviors; in fact, everything we do in life. This imprint is physically imparted onto our DNA when it first forms chemically in that single cell that will later become an individual being.

When we are first stimulated by The Universe, using celestiophysics, we are then given a map of destiny that propels us through life. Some of us follow this map without much thought. Others, like me, question it each day and consciously make a choice whether to follow that map or go "off-map" and do something that we were not initially programmed to do.

These thoughts bring me to my personal philosophy, *Subism.* It holds that the human subconscious is direct communication with The Universe, and that celestial bodies (all forms of matter, energy and unknown entities) directly and indirectly influence all life on earth.

The philosophers of old weren't familiar with celestiophysics, so they formulated their own ideas about how humans operate and function, and what makes us do the things we do.

I do not subscribe to or practice the philosophies of others, because they are all inaccurate, misleading and often destructive. Those people were completely ignorant of how The Universe actually works.

They based their life's work on false assumptions that built an unsteady foundation, a mountain of detritus millions of people have followed and worshiped for millennia. It takes years of study to appreciate this fact.

I suggest that we humans do all the things we do because of the strong, inexorable influences of celestiophysics. Of course, we now know that our kahuni play a huge role in our actions and behaviors. One must wonder how The Universe affects these tiny creatures, which in turn deeply affect our lives.

Use Your Subconscious to Understand Yourself and Accomplish Your Goals in Life

How?

Dreams and dreaming.

Sometimes you may not recall a dream, but your subconscious is actively dreaming, sending little (and giant) messages up to your conscious self to do certain things, avoid other things.

Dreams are one method the CHILD uses to communicate with your conscious self. Interestingly, when your CHILD presents a dream to you, it does so in very rudimentary language, in the language of a child.

We dream in metaphors and symbols and motifs, not in complete film-like visions. This method of communication is as old as The Universe itself and is very effective. One must learn to accurately interpret the messages before any meaningful action can be taken.

Our CHILD only knows one method of talking to our conscious self, and that is in the language of a child, a small voice that expresses itself using little vignettes that represent small words and actions. I've never heard of anyone dreaming in the language of an adult. Never.

If someone tells you that they do in fact dream this way, it's not a deep-sleep dream but a lucid dream, one you actually control because you're partly conscious and are speaking or visualizing in the language of an adult. Again, one must be at least partially conscious during lucid dreaming.

Accurately Interpreting Your Dreams

During a very difficult time in my life some years back, I had a recurring dream: I was sitting in a bus filled with other people. I wasn't talking or interacting with anyone, just sitting alone and minding my own business.

Then the bus suddenly filled with water, as if we'd just plunged into the middle of an ocean. No one around me moved an inch or spoke anything to me or to each other. They all just sat there as the bus filled with water. I looked around, saw stone-cold faces on my fellow passengers, and tried frantically to get out.

And then the dream went lucid, where I could actually manipulate the dream in a semi-conscious state. I changed the dream so I got out of that sinking bus, drove to my fave restaurant in LA, and drowned myself in many craft beers. Much better way of drowning, you ask me.

Since I had already known that my CHILD was responsible for communicating with me, I then figured out a way to interpret what it was trying to tell me. I didn't get it at first, so the dream stayed with me each night for a week or so, until I woke up and listened better.

To interpret my dream, which was in the absurdly simple patois of a child, I used the thoughts, ideas and words of a four year old. When I used this method, interpreting the dream in a child's voice, the dream became clear: "I can't get out and no one will help me. I have to do it on my own." Sounds silly or even simplistic, but it is accurate.

The very day I made this discovery, my life at that time changed dramatically. Allow me to share with you what actually happened to bring on the dream: I had just gone through a painful breakup with my girlfriend and was depressed.

The friends we had when we were together all became her friends, and I was left with no one to talk and share my thoughts with, or to grieve with, let alone get some help from.

The dream told me that I was in a world of hurt and no one was coming to my aid, even when I actively asked for help. In the real world, I was on my own.

I have a term for that: yoyo, which means "you're on your own" when things get really tough for you. I was yoyo for a long time, until I realized what was actually happening, then when I figured out my temporary predicament, I was able to change how I thought, how I acted, and consequently the actions I took to climb out of that dark hole, from inside that sinking bus. It was all in how I viewed it, and so I changed my values, my thoughts.

My CHILD knew what was going on all along and it tried to tell me, using the only language it knew—the small, yet significant, language of a sweet babe.

Now That We Know We Have This Special Gift Inside Us, What's Next?

The first thing I recommend: learn how to feed it properly, to nurture it. You would do this with a human child, wouldn't you? Your CHILD is even more important. It's the entity within yourself that guides you through every moment of your entire life. How could you not want to nurture such a special being?

Your CHILD is energetic and rambunctious, has a voracious appetite for new adventures and actions, so get out in the world and do stuff. Travel to new places, meet new people, eat new foods, explore new vistas.

If you cannot afford to go to Europe or Africa, then explore your own town or city, or maybe drive to the next city or state and see what's up there. If those things are not in your current budget, then find a way to make it happen, now that you know your subconscious needs these things.

Your CHILD loves to run and jump and play around, so get out and exercise your body, even if it's a long walk or hike. If you're going to be a sedentary writer, then your CHILD will eventually rebel.

Yes, I do know some overweight writers who do well, but they don't last too long. Unfortunately, they die young and the being that dies first is their CHILD.

This explains in part how people sometimes grow cold and distant, and they lose their humanity. In reality, they're losing the most important part of them—their subconscious. They are also losing the ability to communicate with the most important entity in their lives: The Universe.

The child inside you needs stimulation, and the world around you provides just that, so please take full advantage of your atmosphere and make it a daily routine to get out of your office and home and see different and stimulating sites, absorb what you sense all around you, roll in the grass, get dirty and make mud pies . . . something cool.

There's a new movement out there that is telling all of us to "ground" our self with the earth. Actually get down on the bare ground and let it touch your skin.

Mother Earth is one giant healing mechanism, so find out more about grounding and then implement your new-found knowledge.

What else? Take trips to local stores, shops, museums, businesses that produce something interesting to see designed or in the process of being built. Feed your imagination 'til its cup runneth over. There are no penalties for overfilling. When your CHILD has had enough, she will tell you.

Go to shows, films, performances and watch the beautiful artwork of people who are just like you: they have a dream, they design and build it, then they do whatever it takes to implement it.

Seeing the art of others is inspiring on all levels, especially when they're actually creating it. Go to the local hardware store and look at all the tools and items that are used to build things. Visit a restaurant and see how they prepare their meals.

What a grand experience to observe artists designing and building artwork! It's not unlike what I do when I create my own work, be it an article or a book. In fact, watching other artists may be the most inspiring thing you can witness for yourself when you go out on these excursions.

I love watching glass-blowers. Especially the truly great ones who produce the world's finest artisan glasswork, those Murano artists in Italy. Wao, they're amazing to watch.

When I'm done witnessing worldclass art in motion, I leave with an all-body tingle. What an inspiration!

How Do You Listen to Your CHILD When It Speaks to You?

First, let's consider when your CHILD is actually trying to communicate with you. An example: you're sitting in a chair, writing away and you get this nagging voice inside your head that says you need a small pillow at your lower back.

Don't ignore it. This is your subconscious telling you something: I want to feel comfortable when I share something important with you. That's like a message from the highest power in The Universe.

Those little voices that creep up at all times of the day and night are your CHILD trying to tell you something. Listen to those voices. When you hear the calling of your subconscious, please pay attention to what it is trying to say, then, provided the command is a reasonable one, please act on it.

Once you start listening to your CHILD, she will say, "Thank you for listening to me!"

And, from that point forward, if you continue to listen to your subconscious, she will give you more and more great knowledge and information that will not only enhance your life, but also teach you The Laws of Creation and how to use them in everyday life.

Communicating with your CHILD is not that challenging. Again, if it tells you to do something and you do it, then you're effectively communicating with her. Keep doing it.

And when you go to bed at night (or during the day, depending on your lifestyle and schedule), ask out loud and write down some questions or topics you want her to mull over. The more you listen to her, the more she will respond and provide the information you need.

You can train her to give you more and more information by asking questions, writing them down, then sleeping on them. Keep asking the same questions over and over until you get what you want or need.

When asking questions or asking for assistance or help (yes, there is a difference!), please be kind to your subconscious. Remember, it is a child and understands when you are being impatient or downright tedious.

You know how people say to treat yourself kindly and gently? They're really saying you should be kind and gentle to the most important creature inside your head: your subconscious.

The reason I suggest you say what you want out loud is because when you speak it and hear your own words, your brain stores and processes that information in different areas, which work in unison to come to your aid.

When you physically write it down, that too is stored and processed in another part of your brain. When you read your own words, that is also stored and processed in yet a different part of your brain.

These working areas are also complex computing centers that help to enhance what you desire and wish for, and they help your CHILD make those wishes and dreams come true. Each reinforces the other that becomes a multiplicative effect: it strengthens all bonds and allows for growth and further learning.

Training your CHILD involves all the above steps, plus actively talking to it, and not just before you go to sleep. You can have meaningful conversations with her, not only asking questions but also asking for guidance and assistance.

The more you communicate with her, the more she responds and with better and more relevant information to help and guide you accurately.

The only time my CHILD has failed me is when I have ignored her. That fact, in itself, I find fascinating and compelling. My CHILD has never steered me in the wrong or in a negative direction. Ever.

When I've chosen to go off-map, then sometimes I've gotten into trouble. Yes, I've learned a lot from those experiential experiences, especially when off-map, but I've also paid a steep price for venturing off my universal path of destiny.

Talking With The Individual Components of Your CHILD

It takes time and effort, and you can do it. I've often consulted my Logic element to get an objective view on a particular subject. And when I've needed to discuss something about my love life, I've talked mostly to my Heart.

Having five separate ultra-complex computer modules inside your head is like having a team of experts at your beck and call. You must treat that team nicely and with great respect or they will ignore you and your queries.

Your CHILD will never be vengeful and send you down a wrong path; only your conscious self does that. The worst you can expect from your subconscious is silence, and that is the most crushing thing that could happen to your beautiful mind, not having the backing of one of the mightiest beings in The Universe.

When your CHILD fails to talk to you or communicate with you, something is very wrong. Remember that she is just that: a child, so she needs special attention.

Like I said, she will never steer you wrong, but she may get pouty and ignore you. If she does, ask what's going on. When you go to bed, write down that question, plus a few others: Are you okay? Have I done anything to make you ignore me? What am I doing wrong here? How can I get back on track? Will you please assist me?

The times I've had my CHILD go silent, they were when I was not treating myself well. Be kind and gentle to yourself, and your CHILD will thank you in ways you cannot even imagine now.

Your CHILD Will Be Your Guide And Mentor In CrossFit

Allow your subconscious to guide you on your CrossFit journey, and you will discover a new set of friends, mentors and colleagues—your CHILD. I always listen to my own CHILD and have never been steered wrong by it. The only time I've failed in some action is when I ignored my subconscious.

CrossFit is probably one of the most challenging routines you will experience in middle age. If you've not been active much over the past 10-20 years, then it will be a struggle for the first year. That's where I was when I started, so I know it can be done.

Each night I asked my subconscious one question or posed a single dilemma, hoping I would get an answer the next day. Sometimes it came, sometimes it took days, weeks. But I eventually got it.

The biggest revelation has been the poor health of my kahuni. Now that I listened better to my CHILD about it, I am taking steps to adjust my intensity, frequency and duration of CrossFit exercises.

I was trying to do too much, too soon, and was frustrated at my lack of progress in the beginning when I did a bootcamp before CrossFit.

My CHILD told me to jump right into CrossFit and I did. It later told me to experiment with various routines, which I still do.

Unfortunately, most won't consider this chapter, let alone study their own subconscious. It's a bit "out there," I know.

My wish for you is that you give it a try, see what happens. I also wish you will discover a whole new world inside your own brain and body, one that calls for you to study it further.

If you're like me, you will not only be pleasantly surprised at what you learn, but shocked at finding a mentor that knows you better than anyone and can advise you on just about anything. It's also a blast to do experiments every few days, asking your subconscious a questions before you sleep and seeing what happens the next morning.

For CrossFit, I ask myself each night: "Am I working too hard for my body?"

In the morning, I am presented with my answer. Most of the time it's a no answer so I proceed with my exercise plans. When it's a yes, I cut back on my exercise routine that day.

So far, using this simple technique of employing my subconscious, I have not been disappointed. But then again I've been practicing this for many years.

On the flip side, I am still working on it with my diet. The only reason I cannot yet adhere to a good healthful diet is because that demon voice inside my kahuni is overriding my subconscious voice.

It's sometimes distressing to know my kahuni is more powerful than my own subconscious. Then again, it is revealing that such a superorgan like the kahuni has great powers. I wonder how I can harness those powers and create a new and better me?

Like I said, I'm a work in progress.

So are you. . . .

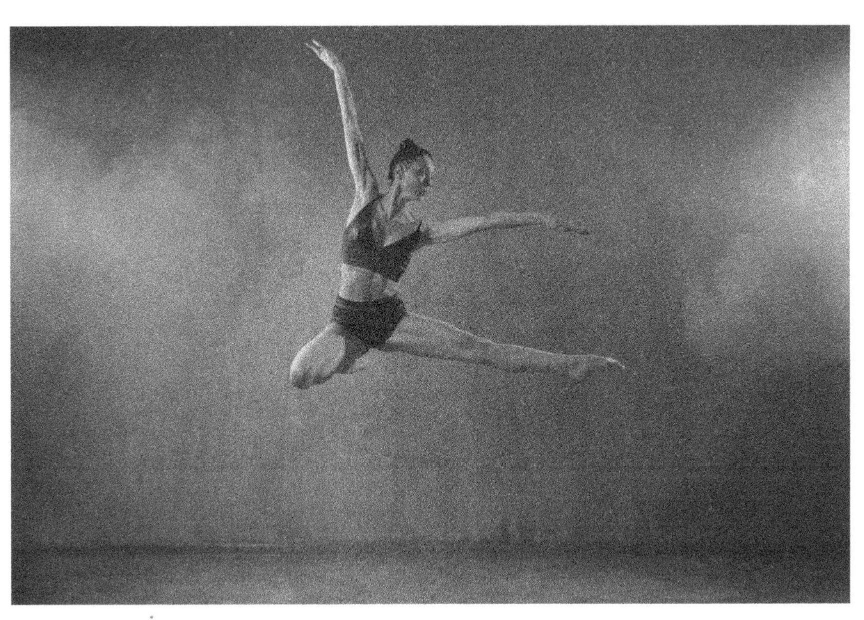

14

Self-Motivation and CrossFit

> "In ten years, my goal is to have 100 million people doing CrossFit."
>
> —Eric Roza
>
> Leader, @CrossFit

You don't have to be a seasoned athlete to do CrossFit. I'm gonna say that again: You don't have to be a seasoned athlete to do CrossFit. Yes, it is a sport and it's sometimes performed at a very high level by some pretty impressive world-class athletes.

And it is also performed by some very ordinary ex-potato-couchers, aka slackletes, like me who never even dreamed of squatting 365 lbs., deadlifting 350 lbs., or doing tabatas til I melted into the floor.

CrossFit is performed by beautiful, energetic age-60+ souls who had previously been stay-at-home moms, overworked lawyers, factory workers with serious injuries, UPS drivers, insurance salespersons, Baskin-Robbins ice cream dippers with carpel-tunnel syndrome, floor installers with back issues, fighter pilots etc.

Word of mouth is still the best form of PR because the information comes from trusted sources. CrossFit Leader Eric Roza says that mothers at his box in Boulder, Colorado bring in more new crossfitters than the coaches do. I'll betcha those mothers are more interested in *exercising* than training. Just a thot.

If you need a little nudge, please consider these helpful mental traits well-adjusted children demonstrate every day. I include them here because as we grow old we often forget the lessons learned as a child. Maybe we should try being a kid again.

These positive traits are based on years of observing some of Amy Morin's patients in psychotherapy. She's a brilliant Licensed Clinical Social Worker, or LCSW, and is my hero!

1. ***They empower themselves*** saying positive things like, "All I can do is try my best," "Act confident," "I'm good enough," "I choose to be happy today."
2. ***They adapt to change*** by articulating their thoughts and emotions, and accurately describing how they feel in that moment.
3. ***They know when to say no.*** Parents help them find polite but firm ways to say no to anyone.
4. ***They own their mistakes*** by learning how to accept defeat and to move on smartly without negative feelings.
5. ***They celebrate the successes of other people*** by saying positive things about them, and congratulating others on doing well.
6. ***They fail and try again*** by learning what went wrong, and not making the same mistake again. Instead, they find new solutions.
7. ***They persist*** even though they don't feel like it.

My gentle suggestion. Though I said it before, it bears repeating: just get to your nearest CrossFit box and begin your new life. I'd also recommend that you see your primary-care physician and get a thorough blood workup and urinalysis to know your current baseline and biomarkers. And don't forget the gut microbe analysis.

Then visit a chiropractor and have them examine your spine and muscles. Unless you have some devastating disease or illness, you can do CrossFit. I was a wreck when I started and now I'm a new man.

Trust me: you do not need any books to start CrossFit and begin your journey to health and happiness.

61 Is The New 41 may be the exception, now that I think on it.

You do not need instructional videos to start CrossFit. You do not need years of preparation just to start CrossFit and enjoy its benefits. Besides, if you took all the advice about stretching and lifting for muscles and joints, you'd need 250 hours in a day. Who has that kinda time?

Please trust me: all you need is a reasonably healthy body, mind, and spirit, and a deep passion to change your life and feel great in all respects.

After that, all you need to do is *show up*.

Remember: you don't have to train at an elite level; you can simply do what I and thousands of others now do: *exercise*!

Oh, it might be cool if you adopted the seven traits seen in mentally and emotionally strong children, too. After all, the child in me wrote this storybook just for you.

So get out there and crossfit yourself to health and well-being. Spread the word and tell others that CrossFit has a new meaning, motto and purpose:

Exercising is the new training!

CrossFit is the new c-word!

61 is the new 41!

"This is all the motivational hoo-haw you need to crossfit yourself to health and well-being, to a new and better *You*."

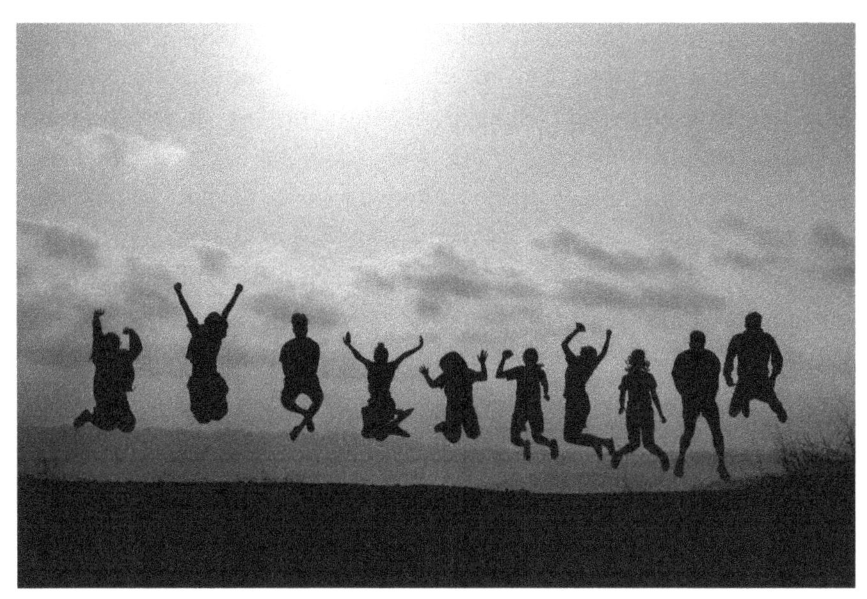

A BIG-ASS THANK-YOU!

Many beautiful souls contributed to this story. I couldn't possibly name them all because they've come and gone from my life over the decades. Thousands who shaped me into the Me of today. Thank you!

In my youth, I was heavily influenced on all levels by a woman whose name shall remain hidden. I saw her at parties my parents took me to in the '60s, when I would be let loose in some neighbor's house while the grown-ups played and partied.

That woman caught me sneakin' around someone's drawers and closets, as I indulged in German and Italian magazines not meant for a nine year old. Near tears with fright and embarrassment, I stopped, now in a frozen state, while she touched my cheek and told me to sit down.

She then said I have two choice in life: one, you can get married and have kids and a nice house . . . *or*, you can have a ***grand*** life of adventure and travel and good people. And good food, too.

With all my heart, mind and soul, I thank this lovely woman-wizard who set me on a glorious path.

Luckily, I was blessed by top-notch professionals whose great writings, wisdom and helpful suggestions greatly improved this book: Karen Brown (film producer), Austin Heaton (HeatonMinded.com), Coach Patrick Higgins (CrossFit Coach), Stew Smith (Navy SEAL and author).

Special thank-yous to Dr. Nick Wignall (NickWignall.com), Dr. Christopher Bergland (read his articles on PsychologyToday.com), Amy Morin, LCSW (AmyMorinLCSW.com) and a few other souls who chose to remain anonymous.

A big thank-you to elite CrossFit athletes Dave Hippensteel and Armando Besne, both of whom contributed their time and effort and shared their stories about what it takes to train after age 61 and beyond. Some of you will want to train instead of exercise. I hope these men's stories will inspire you.

CrossFit X is well represented by Rachel G, Lynda C and Bobby T, all of whom shared deep moving stories about their personal struggles with life and CrossFit. Choosing to exercise for life is ingrained in their souls. Hopefully, you will be stirred by their anecdotes and words of inspiration.

My coach, Patrick Higgins, is the man who made me fall in love with CrossFit and personal training. He's also a pastor who loves people and life, and it shows all the time. The day he blasted Bruno Mars' Perm on the sound system changed my life. Again. I used Bruno as background inspiration when writing much of this book.

Coach Higgins knows more about CrossFit than most, especially those techniques to work the unsung hero stabilizer muscles in the shoulder and core. Soon as he showed those to me, I discovered a new love for exercising, in general. I had no idea that these little muscles lurked beneath the other major muscles that get all the good press. I'm better and stronger because of his worldclass instruction.

I thank all the scientists, physicians, medical and healthcare practitioners, mental-health professionals, and amateur practitioners who contributed books, articles, papers, videos, talks, and phone and email chats. Without their wealth of knowledge, this book would never have been conceived.

There is a growing community of self-taught scientists who are curious, energetic, enthusiastic and determined to study and learn all about the human body. The kahuni offers these people the golden opportunity to unleash human brain power on this burgeoning field of study.

We may not read their work in established scientific and medical books and journals or hear them speak at conferences, but eventually their work will get out. When it does, we will somehow discover it and use it to our benefit.

As I stated before, I pray they are able to perform good research that benefits all before it's too late, i.e. before pharmaceutical companies put a halt to "amateur" and "personal" research in favor of huge profits.

Regardless of the obstacles, life *always* finds a way.

Thank you to John R and Leil G, two athletes who continue to inspire me on my CrossFit journey!

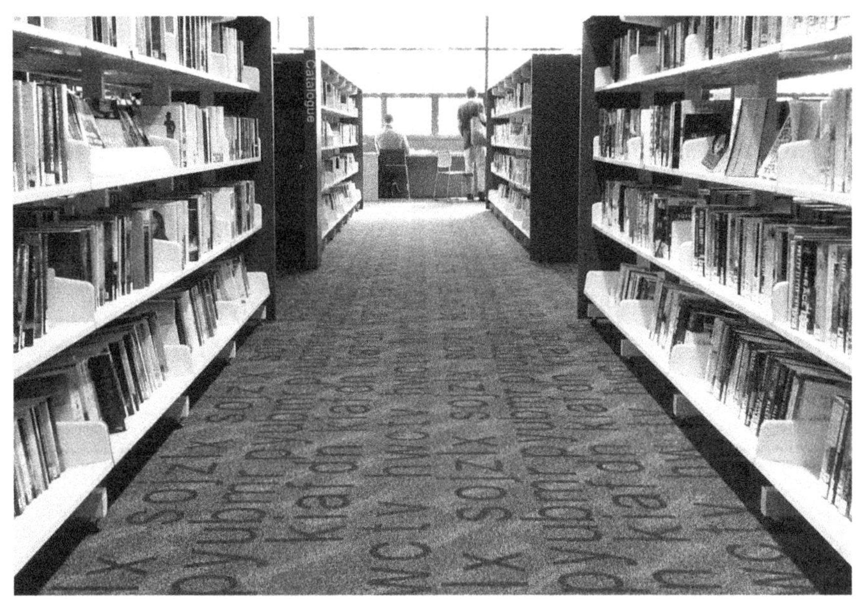

REFERENCES

When doing research for this book, I read hundreds of books, scientific articles and papers, and consulted with several experts. Each piece of information led me to dozens more. At some point, I needed to say *stop* so I could finish writing the book, though it was always tempting to add "just one more important item."

Thankfully, the 61 year old in me took over and allowed reason and rationality to eclipse passion and exuberance.

By far the most important topic of my book is the gut microbiome, your kahuni. I spent countless days reading well into the wee hours, and just as I thought I'd learned a lot, I discovered something entirely new. Or something that contradicted previous information.

Contradictions, objections and refutations always meant that I got to look into the subject much further. In a few cases, I ended up in a stalemate because of the paucity of good data and research results.

The hardest job when doing research is knowing what is good, accurate science and what is bad science. I listened to my subconscious the entire time, and ended up discarding many articles and papers.

Still, in each of the following pieces, I did find at least one small bit of useful information, though some of the experimental and statistical methods were suspect or just plain faulty. Again, even with these faults, there was at least some useful information I feel you should be aware of, things worthy of further study.

I pray the articles and papers I included here are some use to you, as you study and learn for yourself. All articles and papers are in alphabetical order by author. The subject of each paper is clearly expressed in the title.

Sorry about this: I chose not to categorize the pieces because many of the articles and papers could've been placed into multiple categories. I'm afraid you'll have to do a little work on your own. Hint: the majority of these items are about the kahuni.

If I have steered you in the wrong direction with my selections, I deeply apologize. In the least, they should provide you a springboard that launches you into a new realm of research in many different areas, and stimulates you to improve your health and well-being on your long and prosperous CrossFit journey.

Remember: no one said this would be easy.

Allen JM et al. (2018). Exercise Alters Gut Microbiota Composition and Function in Lean and Obese Humans. *Medicine and Science in Sports Exercise*. 50(4):747-757.

Adams DH, Eksteen B and Curbishley SM (2008). Immunology of the gut and liver: a love/hate relationship. *Gut* 57:838–48.

Althoff T et al. (2017). Large-scale physical activity data reveal worldwide activity inequality. *Nature* 547:336-339.

Arpaia N et al. (2013). Metabolites produced by commensal bacteria promote peripheral regulatory T-cell generation. *Nature* 504:451–5.

Arthur JC et al. (2012). Intestinal inflammation targets cancer-inducing activity of the microbiota. *Science* 338:120–3.

Barnich N, Denizot J and Darfeuille-Michaud AE (2013). E coli-mediated gut inflammation in genetically predisposed Crohn's disease patients. *Pathologie Biologie* (Paris) 61:e65–9.

Benjamin JL et al. (2011). Randomised, double-blind, placebo-controlled trial of fructo-oligosaccharides in active Crohn's disease. *Gut* 60:923–9.

Bergland C (2012). The Neurochemicals of Happiness. https://www.psychologytoday.com/us/blog/the-athletes-way/201211/the-neurochemicals-happiness. Accessed and vetted 01 March 2021.

Bergland C (2021). Short on Time? HIIT Workouts May Boost Brain Power Swiftly. https://www.psychologytoday.com/us/blog/the-athletes-way/202105/short-time-hiit-workouts-may-boost-brain-power-swiftly. Accessed and vetted 19 May 2021.

Bergland C (2021). 3 Reasons Real-Life Social Support Is Best for Mental Health. https://www.psychologytoday.com/us/blog/the-athletes-way/202105/3-reasons-real-life-social-support-is-best-mental-health. Accessed and vetted 10 May 2021.

Bergland C (2021). Runner's High Isn't the Only Way to Hack Mu-Opioid Receptors. https://www.psychologytoday.com/us/blog/the-athletes-way/202104/runner-s-high-isn-t-the-only-way-hack-mu-opioid-receptors. Accessed and vetted 24 April 2021.

Bergland C (2021). 6 Reasons to Make HIIT Workouts Part of Your Weekly Routine. https://www.psychologytoday.com/us/blog/the-athletes-way/202104/6-reasons-make-hiit-workouts-part-your-weekly-routine. Accessed and vetted 22 April 2021.

Bergland C (2021). Why 43 Minutes of Cardio a Day May Help Keep the Doctor Away. https://www.psychologytoday.com/us/blog/the-athletes-way/202104/why-43-minutes-cardio-day-may-help-keep-the-doctor-away. Accessed and vetted 19 April 2021.

Bergland C (2021). 2 Ways Cardio Workouts May Help Aging Brains Stay Healthy. https://www.psychologytoday.com/us/blog/the-athletes-way/202104/2-ways-cardio-workouts-may-help-aging-brains-stay-healthy. Accessed and vetted 05 April 2021.

Bergland C (2021). How Staying Physically Fit May Help Kids' Executive Functions. https://www.psychologytoday.com/us/blog/the-athletes-way/202103/how-staying-physically-fit-may-help-kids-executive-functions. Accessed and vetted 29 March 2021.

Bergland C (2021). Want to Sleep Better Tonight? A Single Bout of Cardio May Help. https://www.psychologytoday.com/us/blog/the-athletes-way/202103/want-sleep-better-tonight-single-bout-cardio-may-help. Accessed and vetted 29 March 2021.

Bergland C (2021). Sustaining Daily Activity Levels May Offset Depression Risk. https://www.psychologytoday.com/us/blog/the-athletes-way/202103/sustaining-daily-activity-levels-may-offset-depression-risk. Accessed and vetted 12 March 2021.

Bjornsson E et al. (2005). Intestinal permeability and bacterial growth of the small bowel in patients with primary sclerosing cholangitis. *Scandinavian Journal of Gastroenterology* 40:1090–4.

Bluher M. (2010). The distinction of metabolically 'healthy' from 'unhealthy' obese individuals. *Current Opinion in Lipidology* 21:38–43.

Blumenthal JA et al. (1999). Effects of exercise training on older patients with major depression. *Archives of Internal Medicine* 159: 2349-2356.

BodySmart Health Solutions (2021). Tight and Sore: maybe you are deficient in magnesium? https://www.bodysmart.com.au/health-tips/tight-and-sore-maybe-you-are-deficient-in-magnesium. Accessed and vetted 18 April 2021.

Boleij A, Tjalsma H. (2013). The itinerary of Streptococcus gallolyticus infection in patients with colonic malignant disease. *The Lancet Infectious Diseases* 13:719–24.

Bonnet M et al. (2014). Colonization of the human gut by E. coli and colorectal cancer risk. *Clinical Cancer Research* 20:859–67.

Bourassa M et al. (2016). Butyrate, neuroepigenetics and the gut microbiome: Can a high fiber diet improve brain health? *Neuroscience Letters* 625:56-63.

Brush CJ et al. (2020). A Randomized Trial of Aerobic Exercise for Major Depression: Examining Neural Indicators of Reward and Cognitive Control as Predictors and Treatment Targets. *Psychological Medicine* 24:1-11.

Campbell S and Wisniewski PJ (2017). Exercise is a novel promoter of intestinal health and microbial diversity. *Exercise and Sport Sciences Reviews* 45(1): 41-47.

Campbell S et al. (2016). The effect of diet and exercise on intestinal integrity and microbial diversity in mice. *The Public Library of Science | One* 11(3): 1-17.

Carbonero F et al. (2012). Microbial pathways in colonic sulfur metabolism and links with health and disease. *Frontiers in Physiology* 3:448.

Carek PJ, Laibstain SE and Carek SM (2011). Exercise for the treatment of depression and anxiety. *The International Journal of Psychiatry in Medicine* 41:15-28.

Cat, LA (2019). The decade of the microbiome. https://www.forbes.com/sites/linhanhcat/2019/12/31/decade-of-the-microbiome. Accessed and vetted 13 April 2021.

Centers for Disease Control and Prevention. https://www.cdc.gov/drugresistance/pdf/threats-report/clostridioides-difficile-508.pdf. Accessed and vetted 24 March 2021.

Chalder M et al. (2012). Facilitated physical activity as a treatment for depressed adults: randomised controlled trial. *The British Medical Journal* 344:e2758.

Chatsko, M (2019). Will the gut microbiome change medicine? Wall Street isn't convinced. https://www.fool.com/investing/2019/09/17/will-the-gut-microbiome-change-medicine-wall-stree.aspx. Accessed and vetted 15 April 2021.

Chekroud AM (2017). Bigger data, harder questions—opportunities throughout mental health care. *Journal of the American Medical Association Psychiatry* 74:1183-1184.

Chen HM et al. (2013). Decreased dietary fiber intake and structural alteration of gut microbiota in patients with advanced colorectal adenoma. *The American Journal of Clinical Nutrition* 97(5):1044-52.

Claesson MJ et al. (2012). Gut microbiota composition correlates with diet and health in the elderly. *Nature* 488:178–84.

Clarke G et al. (2014). Minireview: gut microbiota: the neglected endocrine organ. *Molecular Endocrinology* 28:1221–38.

Clemente, JC et al. (2012). The impact of the gut microbiota on human health: an integrative view. *Cell* 148:1258–1270.

Clifford MN (2004). Diet-derived phenols in plasma and tissues and their implications for health. *Planta Medica* 70:1103–14.

Colman RJ and Rubin DT (2014). Fecal microbiota transplantation as therapy for inflammatory bowel disease: a systematic review and meta-analysis. *Journal of Crohn's and Colitis* 8:1569–81.

Cooney G (2013). Exercise for depression. *Journal of Evidence-Based Medicine* 6:307-308

Cooney G, Dwan K and Mead G (2014). Exercise for depression. *Journal of the American Medical Association* 311:2432-2433.

Cornely OA et al. (2012). Treatment of first recurrence of Clostridium difficile infection: fidaxomicin versus vancomycin. *Clinical Infectious Diseases* 55(suppl 2):s154-s161.

Cotillard A et al. (2013). Dietary intervention impact on gut microbial gene richness. *Nature* 500:585–8.

Cryan, J. F. et al. (2019). The Microbiota-Gut-Brain Axis. *Physiological Reviews* 99:1877–2013.

Cuevas-Sierra A et al. (2019). Diet, Gut Microbiota, and Obesity: Links with Host Genetics and Epigenetics and Potential Applications. *Advances in Nutrition* 10(suppl_1):S17-S30.

Cully M (2019). Microbiome therapeutics go small molecule. *Nature Reviews Drug Discovery* 18:569–572.

D'Angelo S and Donini L (2020). The relationship between microbiota and exercise. *Sport Science* 14 Supplement 1:24-29.

David LA et al. (2014). Diet rapidly and reproducibly alters the human gut microbiome. *Nature* 505:559–63.

Davies YK et al. (2008). Long-term treatment of primary sclerosing cholangitis in children with oral vancomycin: an immunomodulating antibiotic. *Journal of Pediatric Gastroenterology and Nutrition* 47:61–7.

de Aguiar Vallim TQ, Tarling EJ and Edwards PA. (2013). Pleiotropic roles of bile acids in metabolism. *Cell Metabolism* 17:657–69.

De Moor MHM et al. (2006). Regular exercise, anxiety, depression and personality: a population-based study. *Preventive Medicine* 42: 273-279.

Denou E et al. (2016). High-intensity exercise training increases the diversity and metabolic capacity of the mouse distal gut microbiota during diet-induced obesity. *American Journal of Physiology, Endocrinology and Metabolism*. 310(11):E982-93.

de Sire A et al. (2020). Gut-joint axis: the role of physical exercise on gut microbiota modulation in older people with osteoarthritis. *Nutrients* 12(2):574.

Dignass A et al. (2012). Second European evidence-based consensus on the diagnosis and management of ulcerative colitis part 2: current management. *Journal of Crohn's and Colitis* 6:991–1030.

Dreher D (2015). How to see yourself more clearly. https://www.psychologytoday.com/us/blog/your-personal-renaissance/201505/how-see-yourself-more-clearly. Accessed and vetted 01 February 2021.

Duncan SH et al. (2008). Human colonic microbiota associated with diet, obesity and weight loss. *International Journal of Obesity* 32:1720–4.

Erickson AR et al. (2012). Integrated metagenomics/metaproteomics reveals human host-microbiota signatures of Crohn's disease. *The Public Library of Science | One* 7:e49138.

Finlay, B. B. (2020). Are noncommunicable diseases communicable? *Science* 367(6475):250-251.

Flint HJ et al. (2012). The role of the gut microbiota in nutrition and health. *Nature Reviews Gastroenterology Hepatology* 9:577–89.

Food and Drug Administration (2016). Enforcement Policy Regarding Investigational New Drug Requirements for Use of Fecal Microbiota for Transplantation to Treat Clostridium difficile Infection Not Responsive to Standard Therapies. https://www.fda.gov/regulatory-information/search-fda-guidance-documents/enforcement-policy-regarding-investigational-new-drug-requirements-use-fecal-microbiota-0. Accessed and vetted 20 April 2021.

Frank DN et al. (2007). Molecular-phylogenetic characterization of microbial community imbalances in human inflammatory bowel diseases. *Proceedings of the National Academy of Sciences* 104:13780–5.

Friedrich MJ (2017). Depression is the leading cause of disability around the world. *Journal of the American Medical Association* 317: 1517

Gibson GR and Roberfroid MB (1995). Dietary modulation of the human colonic microbiota: introducing the concept of prebiotics. *Journal of Nutrition* 125:1401–12.

Gionchetti P et al. (2003). Prophylaxis of pouchitis onset with probiotic therapy: a double-blind, placebo-controlled trial. *Gastroenterology* 124:1202–9.

Gerasimidis K et al. (2014). Decline in presumptively protective gut bacterial species and metabolites are paradoxically associated with disease improvement in pediatric Crohn's disease during enteral nutrition. *Inflammatory Bowel Diseases* 20:861–71.

Gong, J. et al. (2019). The gut microbiome and response to immune checkpoint inhibitors: preclinical and clinical strategies. *Clinical and Translational Medicine* 8:9.

Gopalakrishnan, V. et al. (2018). Gut microbiome modulates response to anti-PD-1 immunotherapy in melanoma patients. *Science* 359(6371):97-103.

Gubert C et al. (2020). Exercise, diet and stress as modulators of gut microbiota: implications for neurodegenerative diseases. *Neurobiology of Disease* 134:1-16

Hajishengallis G, Darveau RP and Curtis MA (2012). The keystone-pathogen hypothesis. *Nature Reviews Microbiology* 10:717–25.

Han YW et al. (2000). Interactions between periodontal bacteria and human oral epithelial cells: Fusobacterium nucleatum adheres to and invades epithelial cells. *Infection and Immunity* 68:3140–6.

Hansen R, Russell RK, Reiff C, et al. (2012). Microbiota of de-novo pediatric IBD: increased *Faecalibacterium prausnitzii* and reduced bacterial diversity in Crohn's but not in ulcerative colitis. *American Journal of Gastroenterology* 107:1913–22.

Harvey SB et al. (2018). Exercise and the prevention of depression: results of the HUNT cohort study. *American Journal of Psychiatry* 175: 28-36.

Helmink, BA et al. (2019). The microbiome, cancer, and cancer therapy. *Nature Medicine* 25:377–388.

Henao-Mejia J et al. (2012). Inflammasome-mediated dysbiosis regulates progression of NAFLD and obesity. *Nature* 482:179–85.

Hermes GDA, Zoetendal EG and Smidt H (2015). Molecular ecological tools to decipher the role of our microbial mass in obesity. *Beneficial Microbes* 6:61–81.

Herring MP, O'Connor PJ and Disham RK (2010). The effect of exercise training on anxiety symptoms among patients. *Archives of Internal Medicine* 170:321-331.

Hill C et al. (2014). Expert consensus document. The International Scientific Association for Probiotics and Prebiotics consensus statement on the scope and appropriate use of the term probiotic. *Nature Reviews Gastroenterology and Hepatology* 11:506–14.

Hofmann SG et al. (2010). The effect of mindfulness-based therapy on anxiety and depression: a meta-analytic review. *Journal of Consulting and Clinical Psychology* 78:169-183.

Hold GL et al. (2014). Role of the gut microbiota in inflammatory bowel disease pathogenesis: what have we learnt in the past 10 years? *World Journal of Gastroenterology* 20:1192–210.

Hu MX et al. (2020). Exercise Interventions for the Prevention of Depression: A Systematic Review of Meta-Analyses. *BioMed Central Public Health* 20:1255.

Hunter P. (2012). The inflammation theory of disease: The growing realization that chronic inflammation is crucial in many diseases opens new avenues for treatment. *European Molecular Biology Organization Reports* 13(11): 968–970.

Ianiro G. et al. (2014). Role of yeasts in healthy and impaired gut microbiota: the gut mycome. *Current Pharmaceutical Design* 20, 4565–4569.

Jones ML, Martoni CJ and Prakash S (2012). Cholesterol lowering and inhibition of sterol absorption by *Lactobacillus reuteri* NCIMB 30242: a randomized controlled trial. *European Journal of Clinical Nutrition* 66:1234–41.

Karlsson FH et al. (2013). Gut metagenome in European women with normal, impaired and diabetic glucose control. *Nature* 498:99–103.

Kashyap PC et al. (2013). Genetically dictated change in host mucus carbohydrate landscape exerts a diet-dependent effect on the gut microbiota. *Proceedings of the National Academy of Science* 110:17059–64.

Kasubuchi M et al. (2015). Dietary gut microbial metabolites, short-chain fatty acids, and host metabolic regulation. *Nutrients.* 7(4):2839-49.

Kaufman J et al. (2004). Social supports and serotonin transporter gene moderate depression in maltreated children. *Proceedings of the National Academy of Science* 101:17316-17321

Kelly CP (2013). Fecal microbiota transplantation—an old therapy comes of age. *New England Journal of Medicine* 368:474–475.

Klok MD, Jacobsdottir S and Drent ML (2006). The role of leptin and ghrelin in the regulation of food intake and body weight in humans: a review. *World Obesity* 8:1, 21-34.

Knudsen KEB et al. (2018). Impact of Diet-Modulated Butyrate Production on Intestinal Barrier Function and Inflammation. *Nutrients.* 10(10):1499.

Kruis W et al. (2004). Maintaining remission of ulcerative colitis with the probiotic *Escherichia coli* Nissle 1917 is as effective as with standard mesalazine. *Gut* 53:1617–23.

Kvam S et al. (2016). Exercise as a treatment for depression: a meta-analysis. *Journal of Affective Disorders* 202:67-86.

Lata J et al. (2011). Probiotics in hepatology. *World Journal of Gastroenterology* 17:2890–6.

Lau JT et al. (2016). Capturing the diversity of the human gut microbiota through culture-enriched molecular profiling. *Genome Medicine* 8(1):72.

Le Chatelier E et al. (2013). Richness of human gut microbiome correlates with metabolic markers. *Nature* 500:541–6.

Lee IM et al. (2012). Effect of physical inactivity on major non-communicable diseases worldwide: an analysis of burden of disease and life expectancy. *Lancet* 380:219-229

Leonel AJ and Alvarez-Leite JI (2012). Butyrate: implications for intestinal function. *Current Opinion in Clinical Nutrition and Metabolic Care* 15(5):474-9.

Leong C and Zelenitsky S (2013). Treatment Strategies for Recurrent *Clostridium difficile* Infection. *Canadian Journal of Hospital Pharmacy* 66(6):361-368.

Lepage P et al. (2013). A metagenomic insight into our gut's microbiome. *Gut* 62:146–58.

Le Roy T et al. (2013). Intestinal microbiota determines development of non-alcoholic fatty liver disease in mice. *Gut* 62:1787–94.

Lessa FC et al. (2015). Burden of *Clostridium difficile* infection in the United States. *New England Journal of Medicine* 372(9):825-834.

Ley RE et al. (2005). Obesity alters gut microbial ecology. *Proceedings of the National Academy of Sciences* 102:11070–5.

Ley RE et al. (2006). Microbial ecology: human gut microbes associated with obesity. *Nature* 444:1022–3.

Lindsay JO et al. (2006). Clinical, microbiological, and immunological effects of fructo-oligosaccharide in patients with Crohn's disease. *Gut* 55:348–55.

Liu H et al. (2018). Butyrate: A Double-Edged Sword for Health? *Advances in Nutrition* 9(1):21-29.

Louis P et al. (2010). Diversity of human colonic butyrate-producing bacteria revealed by analysis of the butyryl-CoA:acetate CoA-transferase gene. *Environmental Microbiology* 12:304–14.

Lu R et al. (2014). Enteric bacterial protein AvrA promotes colonic tumorigenesis and activates colonic beta-catenin signaling pathway. *Oncogenesis* 3:e105.

Lupp C et al. (2007). Host-mediated inflammation disrupts the intestinal microbiota and promotes the overgrowth of Enterobacteriaceae. *Cell Host and Microbe* 2:204.

Ma YY et al. (2013). Effects of probiotics on nonalcoholic fatty liver disease: a meta-analysis. *World Journal of Gastroenterology* 19:6911–18.

Macfarlane GT and Macfarlane S (2011). Fermentation in the human large intestine: its physiologic consequences and the potential contribution of prebiotics. *Journal of Clinical Gastroenterology* 45 Suppl:S120-7.

Mailing LJ et al. (2019). Exercise and the gut microbiome: a review of the evidence, potential mechanisms, and implications for human health. *Exercise and Sport Sciences Reviews* 47(2):75-85.

Manichanh C et al. (2006). Reduced diversity of faecal microbiota in Crohn's disease revealed by a metagenomic approach. *Gut* 55:205–11.

Marchesi JR et al. (2016). The gut microbiota and host health: a new clinical frontier. *Gut* 65:330-339.

Marchesi JR et al. (2011). Towards the human colorectal cancer microbiome. *The Public Library of Science | One* 6:e20447.

Matthews M (2019). *Bigger Leaner Stronger: The Simple Science of Building the Ultimate Male Body*, 3rd edition. Oculus Publishers, Clearwater.

Matthews M (2019). *Thinner Leaner Stronger: The Simple Science of Building the Ultimate Female Body*. Oculus Publishers, Clearwater.

Mattner J et al. (2011). Liver autoimmunity triggered by microbial activation of natural killer T cells. *Cell Host and Microbe* 3:304–15.

McDonald LC et al. (2018). Clinical practice guidelines for *Clostridium difficile* infection in adults and children: 2017 update by the Infectious Diseases Society of America (IDSA) and Society for Healthcare Epidemiology of America (SHEA). *Clinical Infectious Diseases* 66(7):e1-e48.

Miele L et al. (2009). Increased intestinal permeability and tight junction alterations in nonalcoholic fatty liver disease. *Hepatology* 49:1877–87.

Moayyedi P et al. (2015). Fecal microbiota transplantation induces remission in patients with active ulcerative colitis in a randomized, controlled trial. *Gastroenterology* 149:102–9.e6.

Morgan XC et al. (2012). Dysfunction of the intestinal microbiome in inflammatory bowel disease and treatment. *Genome Biology* 3:R79.

Morishima S et al. (2021). Intensive, prolonged exercise seemingly causes gut dysbiosis in female endurance runners. *Journal of Clinical Biochemistry and Nutrition* 68(3): 253–258.

Muegge BD, Kuczynski J et al. (2011). Diet drives convergence in gut microbiome functions across mammalian phylogeny and within humans. *Science* 332:970–4.

Mukhopadhya I et al. (2011). Detection of Campylobacter concisus and other Campylobacter species in colonic biopsies from adults with ulcerative colitis. *The Public Library of Science | One* 6:e21490.

National Institutes of Health (2019). A review of 10 years of human microbiome research activities at the US National Institutes of Health, Fiscal Years 2007-2016. *Microbiome* 7, 31.

Nelson WW, et al. (2021). Health care resource utilization and costs of recurrent *Clostridioides difficile* infection in the elderly: a real-world claims analysis. *Journal of Managed Care and Specialty Pharmacy* 1-11.

Ng SC et al. (2009). Mechanisms of action of probiotics: recent advances. *Inflammatory Bowel Diseases* 15:300–10.

Nguyen TTT et al. (2018). Cultivable butyrate-producing bacteria of elderly Japanese diagnosed with Alzheimer's disease. *Journal of Microbiology* 56(10):760-771.

Nieman DC and Wentz LM (2019). The compelling link between physical activity and the body's defense system. *Journal of Sport and Health Science* 8:201-217.

Norman JM et al. (2015). Disease-specific alterations in the enteric virome in inflammatory bowel disease. *Cell* 160:447–60.

O'Hara AM and Shanahan F (2006). The gut flora as a forgotten organ. *European Molecular Biology Organization Reports* 7:688–693.

O'Keefe SJ et al. (2015). Fat, fibre and cancer risk in African Americans and rural Africans. *Nature Communications* 6:6342.

Ou J et al. (2013). Diet, microbiota, and microbial metabolites in colon cancer risk in rural Africans and African Americans. *American Journal of Clinical Nutrition* 98:111–20.

Pagnini C et al. (2011). Alteration of local microflora and alpha-defensins hyper-production in colonic adenoma mucosa. *Journal of Clinical Gastroenterology* 45:602–10.

Pande C, Kumar A and Sarin SK (2009). Small-intestinal bacterial overgrowth in cirrhosis is related to the severity of liver disease. *Alimentary Pharmacology and Therapeutics* 29: 1273–81.

Pariente N and York A (2019). Milestones in human microbiota research. https://www.nature.com/immersive/d42859-019-00041-z/index.html. Accessed and vetted 06 April 2021.

Pennisi E (2020). Meet the 'psychobiome': the gut bacteria that may alter how you think, feel, and act. https://www.sciencemag.org/news/2020/05/meet-psychobiome-gut-bacteria-may-alter-how-you-think-feel-and-act. Accessed and vetted 16 April 2021.

Penney N et al. (2020). Investigating the role of diet and exercise in gut microbe-host cometabolism. *mSystems* 5(6):1-16.

Peterson DA et al. (2008). Metagenomic approaches for defining the pathogenesis of inflammatory bowel diseases. *Cell Host and Microbe* 3:417–27.

Pinto Pereira SM, Geoffroy M-C and Power C. (2014). Depressive symptoms and physical activity during 3 decades in adult life: bidirectional associations in a prospective cohort study. *Journal of the American Medical Association Psychiatry* 71:1373-1380

Poole DC et al. (2007). The final frontier: oxygen flux into muscle at exercise outset. *Exercise and Sport Sciences Reviews* 35(4): 166-173.

Prorok-Hamon M et al. (2014). Colonic mucosa-associated diffusely adherent afaC+ *Escherichia coli* expressing lpfA and pks are increased in inflammatory bowel disease and colon cancer. *Gut* 63:761–70.

Qin J et al. (2012). A metagenome-wide association study of gut microbiota in type 2 diabetes. *Nature* 490:55–60.

Queipo-Ortuno MI et al. (2012). Influence of red wine polyphenols and ethanol on the gut microbiota ecology and biochemical biomarkers. *American Journal of Clinical Nutrition* 95:1323–34.

Quraishi SM et al. (2014). Probing the microbiota in PSC: the gut adherent microbiota of PSC-IBD is distinct to that of IBD and controls. *Hepatology* 60:267A.

Rajilic-Stojanovic M and de Vos WM (2014). The first 1000 cultured species of the human gastrointestinal microbiota. *Federal of European Microbiological Societies Microbiology Reviews* 38:996–1047.

Raman M et al. (2013). Fecal microbiome and volatile organic compound metabolome in obese humans with nonalcoholic fatty liver disease. *Clinical Gastroenterology and Hepatology* 11:868–75. e1–3.

Reimann A et al. (2015). Acidic environment activates inflammatory programs in fibroblasts via a cAMP–MAPK pathway. *Biochimica et Biophysica Acta Molecular Cell Research* 1853(2):299-307.

Rethorst CD et al. (2017). Prediction of treatment outcomes to exercise in patients with nonremitted major depressive disorder. *Depression and Anxiety* 34:1116-1122

Rincon D et al. (2014). Oral probiotic VSL#3 attenuates the circulatory disturbances of patients with cirrhosis and ascites. *Liver International* 34:1504–12.

Romero-Corral A et al. (2008). Accuracy of body mass index in diagnosing obesity in the adult general population. *International Journal of Obesity* 32:959–66.

Rosenbaum S, Sherrington C and Tiedemann A (2015). Exercise augmentation compared with usual care for post-traumatic stress disorder: a randomized controlled trial. *Acta Psychiatrica Scandinavica* 131:350-359

Rossen NG et al. (2015). The mucosa-associated microbiota of PSC patients is characterized by low diversity and low abundance of uncultured Clostridiales II. *Journal of Crohn's and Colitis* 9:342–8.

Rossen NG et al. (2015). Findings from a randomized controlled trial of fecal transplantation for patients with ulcerative colitis. *Gastroenterology* 149:110–18.e4.

Rubinstein MR et al. (2013). Fusobacterium nucleatum promotes colorectal carcinogenesis by modulating E-cadherin/beta-catenin signaling via its FadA adhesin. *Cell Host and Microbe* 14:195–206.

Sberro H et al. (2019). Large-scale analyses of human microbiomes reveal thousands of small, novel genes. *Cell* 178, 1245-1259.e14.

Scanlan PD et al. (2008). Culture-independent analysis of the gut microbiota in colorectal cancer and polyposis. *Environmental Microbiology* 10:789–98.

Schuch FB et al. (2016). Exercise as a treatment for depression: a meta-analysis adjusting for publication bias. *Journal of Psychiatric Research* 77:42-51.

Schuch FB et al. (2018). Physical activity and incident depression: a meta-analysis of prospective cohort studies. *American Journal of Psychiatry* 175(7):631-648.

Sears CL and Pardoll DM (2011). Perspective: alpha-bugs, their microbial partners, and the link to colon cancer. *Journal of Infectious Diseases* 203:306–11.

Segata N et al. (2012). Composition of the adult digestive tract bacterial microbiome based on seven mouth surfaces, tonsils, throat and stool samples. *Genome Biology* 13:R42.

Shen J, Zuo ZX and Mao AP (2014). Effect of probiotics on inducing remission and maintaining therapy in ulcerative colitis, Crohn's disease, and pouchitis: meta-analysis of randomized controlled trials. *Inflammatory Bowel Diseases* 20:21–35.

Shen XJ et al. (2010). Molecular characterization of mucosal adherent bacteria and associations with colorectal adenomas. *Gut Microbes* 1:138–47.

Silgailis M (2017). Gut microbe differences between active and sedentary women. https://lactobacto.com/2017/02/14/gut-microbe-differences-between-active-and-sedentary-women/. Accessed and vetted 02 April 2021.

Sivaprakasam S, Prasad PD and Singh N (2016). Benefits of short-chain fatty acids and their receptors in inflammation and carcinogenesis. *Pharmacology and Therapeutics* 164:144-51.

Sokol H et al. (2009). Low counts of Faecalibacterium prausnitzii in colitis microbiota. *Inflammatory Bowel Diseases* 15:1183–9.

Son G, Kremer M and Hines IN (2010). Contribution of gut bacteria to liver pathobiology. *Gastroenterology Research and Practice* 2010:1–13.

Stilling RM et al. (2016). The neuropharmacology of butyrate: The bread and butter of the microbiota-gut-brain axis? *Neurochemistry International* 99:110-132.

Stripling J and Rodriguez M (2018). Current evidence in delivery and therapeutic uses of fecal microbiota transplantation in human diseases—*Clostridium difficile* disease and beyond. *The American Journal of Medical Sciences* 356:424–432.

Swidsinski A et al. (2005). Spatial organization and composition of the mucosal flora in patients with inflammatory bowel disease. *Journal of Clinical Microbiology* 43:3380–9.

Sui SX and Pasco JA . (2020). Obesity and brain function: The brain–body crosstalk. *Medicina* 56(10):49922020

Sui SX, Ridding MC and Hordacre B (2020). Obesity is associated with reduced plasticity of the human motor cortex. *Brain Sciences* 10(9):579.

Sui SX et al. (2021). Skeletal muscle density and cognitive function: a cross-sectional study in men. *Calcified Tissue International* 1-1132020

Sui SX et al. (2020). Skeletal muscle health and cognitive function: a narrative review. *International Journal of Molecular Sciences* 22(1):255.

Sui SX et al. (2020). Muscle strength and gait speed rather than lean mass are better indicators for poor cognitive function in older men. *Scientific Reports* 10(1):1-9.

Tabata I (2019). Tabata training: one of the most energetically effective high-intensity intermittent training methods. *The Journal of Physiological Sciences*, 69:559-572.

Tabibian JH, Talwalkar JA and Lindor KD (2013). Role of the microbiota and antibiotics in primary sclerosing cholangitis. *BioMed Research International* 2013:389537.

Tang WH et al. (2013). Intestinal microbial metabolism of phosphatidylcholine and cardiovascular risk. *New England Journal of Medicine* 368:1575–84.

Tedelind S et al. (2007). Anti-inflammatory properties of the short-chain fatty acids acetate and propionate: a study with relevance to inflammatory bowel disease. *World Journal of Gastroenterology* 13(20):2826-32.

Tembo MC et al (2020). Total Antioxidant Capacity and Frailty in Older Men. *American Journal of Men's Health* 14(5):1557988320946592.

Tembo MC et al. (2020). Prevalence of Frailty in Older Men and Women: Cross-Sectional Data from the Geelong Osteoporosis Study. *Calcified Tissue International* 107(3):220-22912020.

Ten Have M, de Graaf R and Monshouwer K (2011). Physical exercise in adults and mental health status. Findings from the Netherlands Mental Health Survey and Incidence Study (NEMESIS). *Journal of Psychosomatic Research* 71:342-348

Thomas AM et al. (2016). Tissue-Associated Bacterial Alterations in Rectal Carcinoma Patients Revealed by 16S rRNA Community Profiling. *Frontiers in Cellular and Infection Microbiology* 6:179.

Thorkildsen LT et al. (2013). Dominant fecal microbiota in newly diagnosed untreated inflammatory bowel disease patients. *Gastroenterology Research and Practice* 2013:636785.

Tjalsma H et al. (2012). A bacterial driver-passenger model for colorectal cancer: beyond the usual suspects. *Nature Reviews Microbiology* 10:575–82.

Tojo R et al. (2014). Intestinal microbiota in health and disease: role of bifidobacteria in gut homeostasis. *World Journal of Gastroenterology* 20(41):15163-15176.

Toseeb U Brage S Corder K et al. (2014). Exercise and depressive symptoms in adolescents: a longitudinal cohort study. *Journal of the American Medical Association Pediatrics* 168:1093-1100

Totorro J (2018). How lack of magnesium impacts athletes. https://www.thorne.com/take-5-daily/article/how-lack-of-magnesium-impacts-athletes. Accessed and vetted 10 March 2021.

Toups M et al. (2017). Exercise is an effective treatment for positive valence symptoms in major depression. *Journal of Affective Disorders* 209:188-194.

Trachsel J et al. (2016). Function and Phylogeny of Bacterial Butyryl Coenzyme A:Acetate Transferases and Their Diversity in the Proximal Colon of Swine. *Applied and Environmental Microbiology* 82(22):6788-6798.

Trivedi MH et al. (2011). Exercise as an augmentation treatment for nonremitted major depressive disorder: a randomized, parallel dose comparison. *Journal of Clinical Psychiatry* 72:677-684.

Tuohy K, Del Rio D, editors. (2014). *Diet-microbe interactions in the gut. Effects on human health and disease.* Academic Press, London.

Turroni S et al. (2018). Microbiota–Host Transgenomic Metabolism, Bioactive Molecules from the Inside. *Journal of Medicinal Chemistry* 61:47–61.

Tursi A et al. (2010). Treatment of relapsing mild-to-moderate ulcerative colitis with the probiotic VSL#3 as adjunctive to a standard pharmaceutical treatment: a double-blind, randomized, placebo-controlled study. *American Journal of Gastroenterology* 105:2218–27.

van Nood, E. et al. (2013). Duodenal infusion of donor feces for recurrent *Clostridium difficile. New England Journal of Medicine* 368:407–415.

Visconti, A. et al. (2019). Interplay between the human gut microbiome and host metabolism. *Nature Communications* 10:4505.

Vrieze A et al. (2012). Transfer of intestinal microbiota from lean donors increases insulin sensitivity in individuals with metabolic syndrome. *Gastroenterology* 143:913–6.e7.

Walker AW et al. (2011). High-throughput clone library analysis of the mucosa-associated microbiota reveals dysbiosis and differences between inflamed and non-inflamed regions of the intestine in inflammatory bowel disease. *BioMed Central Microbiology* 11:7.

Wang B et al. (2017). The Human Microbiota in Health and Disease. *Engineering* 3:71–82.

Wang L et al. (2019). Natural Products from Mammalian Gut Microbiota. *Trends in Biotechnology* 37:492–504.

Wang T et al. (2012). Structural segregation of gut microbiota between colorectal cancer patients and healthy volunteers. *The ISME Journal* 6(2):320-9.

Wang X, Yang Y and Huycke MM. (2015). Commensal bacteria drive endogenous transformation and tumour stem cell marker expression through a bystander effect. *Gut* 64:459–68.

Warren RL et al. (2013). Co-occurrence of anaerobic bacteria in colorectal carcinomas. *Microbiome* 1:16.

Weir T (2017). Exercise: the next frontier in microbiota research? *Exercise and Sport Sciences Reviews* 45(1):4-5.

Wikoff WR et al. (2009). Metabolomics analysis reveals large effects of gut microflora on mammalian blood metabolites. *Proceedings of the National Academy of Sciences* 106(10):3698-703.

Wilmanski T et al. (2019). Blood metabolome predicts gut microbiome alpha-diversity in humans. *Nature Biotechnology* 37, 1217–1228.

Windey K, De Preter V, Verbeke K. (2012). Relevance of protein fermentation to gut health. *Molecular Nutrition and Food Research* 56:184–96.

World Health Organization, Food and Agricultural Organization of the United Nations. Health and nutritional properties of probiotics in food including powder milk with live lactic acid bacteria. *Food and Agriculture Organization Nutrition Paper* 85.

Wu GD et al. (2011). Linking long-term dietary patterns with gut microbial enterotypes. *Science* 334:105–8.

Wu N et al. (2013). Dysbiosis signature of fecal microbiota in colorectal cancer patients. *Microbial Ecology* 66(2):462-70.

Wu S et al. (2009). A human colonic commensal promotes colon tumorigenesis via activation of T helper type 17T cell responses. *Nature Medicine* 15:1016–22.

Wu X et al. (2010). Molecular characterisation of the faecal microbiota in patients with type II diabetes. *Current Microbiology* 61(1):69-78.

Wylie KM et al. (2012). Emerging view of the human virome. *Translational Research* 160, 283–290.

Yan AW and Schnabl B. (2012). Bacterial translocation and changes in the intestinal microbiome associated with alcoholic liver disease. *World Journal of Hepatology* 4:110–18.

Yan AW et al. (2011). Enteric dysbiosis associated with a mouse model of alcoholic liver disease. *Hepatology* 53:96–105.

Ze X et al. (2013). Some are more equal than others: the role of "keystone" species in the degradation of recalcitrant substrates. *Gut Microbes* 4:236–40.

Zhang M et al. (2009). Pattern extraction of structural responses of gut microbiota to rotavirus infection via multivariate statistical analysis of clone library data. *FEMS Microbiology Ecology* 70(2):21-9.

Zhang Y et al. (2018). Changes in gut microbiota and plasma inflammatory factors across the stages of colorectal tumorigenesis: a case-control study. *BioMed Central Microbiology* 18(1):92.

Zhu L et al. (2013). Characterization of gut microbiomes in nonalcoholic steatohepatitis (NASH) patients: a connection between endogenous alcohol and NASH. *Hepatology* 57:601–9.

Zhu Q et al. (2014). Analysis of the intestinal lumen microbiota in an animal model of colorectal cancer. *The Public Library of Science | One* 9:e90849.

Zoetendal EG et al. (2012). The human small intestinal microbiota is driven by rapid uptake and conversion of simple carbohydrates. *ISME Journal* 6:1415–26.

Zupancic ML et al. (2012). Analysis of the gut microbiota in the old order Amish and its relation to the metabolic syndrome. *The Public Library of Science | One* 7:e43052.

CPSIA information can be obtained
at www.ICGtesting.com
Printed in the USA
LVHW110115230621
690870LV00004B/224